UNFOLDING OUR LIGHT

by the same author

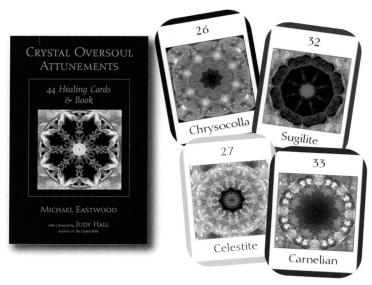

Designed for meditation and contemplation, this set of beautiful cards and accompanying book explore in great depth the spiritual and metaphysical qualities of crystals and how to communicate with the part of the collective consciousness that the crystals represent. Each card is a photographic mandala featuring a different crystal that conveys messages directly into the consciousness of the viewer. The book contains information about crystal healing and meditation practice. Together the cards and the book build a map, representing the shared spiritual and healing potential that these meditations can bring.

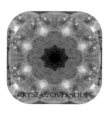

The *Crystal Oversoul Attunements* Cards are also available as an iOS app from iTunes.

UNFOLDING OUR LIGHT

Creating Crystal Mandalas to Awaken and Heal

MICHAEL EASTWOOD

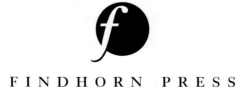

FINDHORN PRESS

First published by Findhorn Press 2013

ISBN 978-1-84409-622-0

British Library Cataloguing-in-Publication Data:
A catalogue record for this book is available from the British Library.

Edited by Michael Hawkins
Cover and interior design by Thierry Bogliolo
Photographs and drawings by Michael Eastwood
Author photography by Marius von Brasch
Printed and bound in the European Union

Published by
Findhorn Press
117-121 High Street
Forres IV36 1AB
Scotland, UK

t +44(0)1309 690582
f +44(0)131 777 2711
e info@findhornpress.com

www.findhornpress.com

Contents

*This book is dedicated to
my beloved husband Marius, my best friend
and traveller through these unfolding times.*

*Also to two of my dearest friends – Lisa
Tenzin-Dolma and Lisa De Malpas Finlay.*

About the Author

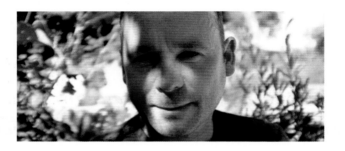

Michael Eastwood is an author and teacher who has specialized in crystal healing for over twenty years. He has facilitated workshops around the world.

He is director of AristiA, a crystal supplier and healing centre in Hampshire.

Michael has been the Chair of the Affiliation of Crystal Healing Organizations (ACHO) since 2009 and is also the current Chair of the Crystal Therapy Council (CTC). He teaches two-year and post-graduate diplomas in crystal healing that take students to the level of qualified practitioners.

Foreword

In this time of rapid transformation, many of us who work to claim remembrance of the ancient wisdom of the crystalline energy will rejoice in this latest book by Michael Eastwood. Here we have the offering of an awakened elder, guide, mystic, teacher and initiator.

Through Michael's personal experience, each Crystal Oversoul speaks directly to us, in many voices, but with the unified authority and presence of the One. They remind us of our vastness, our true Soul potential, and our need to reclaim our ancient Lemurian history.

In Lemuria we lived as our Soul, we used our knowledge and wisdom for the benefit of all. The Earth was purer then and communication between other dimensions and realms was easier, flowing effortlessly; everything was pristine.

In this book, the Crystal Oversouls dare us to remember our original descent into matter, heaven sent, and on a mission as co-creators of this intriguing, magnificent world.

Through Michael's guidance, you will see yourself and the potential to be who your Divine self is meant to be and so much more. You will be guided through dimensional portals, into worlds of indescribable beauty and bliss.

I first met Michael over twenty years ago, we have remained friends, crystal explorers and crystal pioneers ever since. So you can imagine my honour and deep delight when I was asked to write the foreword for this unique book.

The simple truth is, I love this wonderful book, it draws you in from the moment you open it. Michael has an eloquent way with words, his deep insight is based on over twenty years' experience of the crystal kingdom and a lifetime of working with light beings. His work is inspirational and delivered with unique clarity.

I highly recommend it to anyone who seeks a greater understanding of the *Crystal Oversoul*s, attunement, chakras, transpersonal chakras and aura.

Your true remembrance and your destiny await you.

—Hazel Raven.
author of *The Angel Bible* and *Crystal Healing*

Introduction

This book is part of a childhood dream of mine. From early on I felt that there are many beings of otherworldly consciousness living amongst humanity and I knew this to be true because I saw and communicated with two large beings of light that accompanied me and stood besides me during my bed times.

In my room I also saw many other beings apparently not of human origin. These beings had the appearance of fine spherical layers of light and although we did not communicate I sensed that they were benevolent. Over time I started to talk with the light-beings, asked them questions, from typical childhood anxieties to questions of a cosmic nature, and somehow I knew that they were with me on purpose.

They impressed upon me that they originated from star worlds, and sought to comfort, educate and remind me of my own star world heritage. They told me that I, and many others, are here in this lifetime for a specific purpose, that we are ancient multi-dimensional luminous beings that in ancient days came from Lemuria and, before then, the stars.

What I understand now is that, since Lemuria, many of us have been asleep, still incarnating but without our full capacities or knowledge of our vastness. This is mirrored in our chakra and auric layers.

"In Lemuria", they tell me, *"your vastness was reflected through at least ten layers of your aura as well as ten chakras, awakened and fully operational. In this lifetime humanity, as well as all kingdoms of this planet, will awaken from this slumber through an initiation – the like that has not been since since Lemurian times. This initi-*

ation will activate the ten layers of your aura as well as all ten chakras. Through this you and humanity will remember union with the wider universe. This human initiation will be keenly watched by the inner planes as well as other star worlds – it involves them too."

Later in life I started to meet other people who in different ways had received the same message and sensed that something important would happen to them and humanity in this lifetime. I discovered that there are, in fact, many thousands of people who like me carry a similar dream of being ancient beings awakening to a higher purpose. I read the works of two visionaries, Ken Carey's *Starseed Transmissions* and Solara's *The Legend of Altazar* and *Star-Borne*. These two writers and dreamers, especially, inspired me to make a contribution to an emerging new consciousness.

I have been trading, teaching and healing within the field of crystal healing for over twenty five years. Through my work I have sought to marry my childhood dialogues with the light beings within the framework of crystal healing, which led me into researching crystals, the human energy field and chakra system.

In this research I came across many references both in ancient spiritual texts and modern day writers that referred to seven levels of the aura as well as seven chakras, which contradicted the light-beings' information I had received about having at least ten layers to the aura and ten chakra gateways. I started to understand that my work was to explore this subject and ultimately offer a model that reflected my own insight and understanding.

As I was piecing it all together I explored the relationship between crystals and the human aura which led me to a profound experience. It was during this that I met and dialogued with an Oversoul. This eventually led to the publication of *The Crystal*

*Oversoul Attunement*s (Findhorn Press, 2011). The dialogues I had with the Crystal Oversouls became the missing key that unlocked the door that enabled me to understand the ten layers of the aura as well as how to awaken all ten chakras.

This book is the result of my research – a navigation guide through the ten layers of the human aura as well as the ten chakra gateways, supporting us to an awakening into the vast luminous beings that we are. With the help of the crystal kingdom and the Crystal Oversouls, we are ready to expand our light and so this book is titled *Unfolding Our Light*.

This book is also a journey – each layer of the aura and corresponding chakra is approached with a series of attunements that are designed to expand and reorganize our aura and chakras to a wider template befitting the collective initiation of our time.

With such a large and open map we can operate in multi-dimensional awareness with ease, taking our rightful place in the universe. What I offer through this book is a way of making our journey creative, joyful; one that supports our inquisitive nature.

In case you are unfamiliar with the term *Oversoul* I repeat here the account of my first experience with Oversouls as given in the accompanying book for the card deck *The Crystal Oversoul Attunements* (Findhorn Press, 2011):

"My first experience of an Oversoul happened one day when I had started to write about Ajoite. I sat in front of my computer thinking about this particular mineral's healing properties when suddenly I found my awareness shifting and traveling at what seemed like the speed of light out of my body. Somehow whatever was happening to me seemed fine and I trusted in the process, although it was a completely new experience for me. I knew my physical body was sitting in front of the computer and time was moving at its usual speed, but my inner travel seemed to last for ages.

I found myself suddenly arriving at what seemed to be a space outside the earth's atmosphere. There in front of me was an enormous portal or mandala of the most vivid turquoise light. The mandala seemed to be moving inwards and pulling my attention into itself. There was an indescribable sound emanating from deep within its centre. I knew already that this was the oversoul of Ajoite.

Although I had no previous conscious knowledge of what an oversoul was or is, I knew that this presence wanted to tell me its story. I felt drawn inside and my consciousness dissolved into the light.

After what seemed like an age, I found myself back on the outer edges of the mandala, covered in a residual light and full of information. I thanked the presence for my profound experience.

After a while, I was aware of having returned into my physical body, on earth and in front of my computer. I sat for a long time trying to comprehend what had just happened and knew that I would need some time to process my encounter. This same experience happened with each crystal I wrote about, and in time it dawned on me that each one would impress its story and trust in me to share its history."

These encounters were not easy for me. After each one I would feel like I had been electrocuted. In time though, the experience eased as I adjusted to the Oversouls' frequencies.

The colourful mandalas represent as near as possible my impression of each of the crystal Oversoul's consciousness and spirit. I feel that these mandalas convey in a visual form each crystal's personality.

By gazing upon or meditating with them a connection can be made.

To my understanding an Oversoul is the collective soul or

master that all individual crystals in its field will identify and communicate with. When we work thus, for example with an Ajoite, we can communicate with its essential soul, its blueprint, its oversoul.

There is a quote by Ralph Waldo Emerson that encapsulates the oversoul idea:

"We live in succession, in division, in parts, in particles. Meantime within man is the soul of the whole; the wise silence; the universal beauty, to which every part and particle is equally related, the eternal ONE. And this deep power in which we exist and whose beatitude is all accessible to us, is not only self-sufficing and perfect in every hour, but the act of seeing and the thing seen, the seer and the spectacle, the subject and the object, are one. We see the world piece by piece, as the sun, the moon, the animal, the tree; but the whole, of which these are shining parts, is the soul." [1]

One of the many questions I had while writing the oversoul stories was: Why tell their story now? What follows is my interpretation of what they impressed upon me.

"Crystal Oversouls are part of the fabric of cosmic creation. They have their own destiny while at the same time their evolution is inter-linked with our own. The earth is undergoing an immense initiation the like of which has not been seen for thousands of years. This initiation doesn't involve only humanity, all living creatures, but also all the elemental kingdoms. The initiation is of cosmic origin, part of a great turning within the ever-evolving wheels of the cosmos. This turning in evolution involves, amongst other forces, the conscious effort of thousands of like-minded beings. Such beings of immense awareness need to work as one unified consciousness, with the cooperation of the many other kingdoms taking part in the shift.

---

[1] From The Over-Soul in Essays: First Series, 1841

The Crystal Oversouls once worked more closely with humanity. They were highly revered within the temples of Lemuria and subsequent times when communication between the inner planes was stronger. As those times have faded in human memory, humanity has also forgotten its history. The Crystal Oversouls hold keys to our awakening. They did not create these keys but hold them in their essence until such a time when we need reminding. They serve to expand our horizons, to awake to our greatness, to be the beings of light that we are.

As we awaken to who we are we start to see with a much wider perspective using sensory chakras and layers of our energy bodies, long forgotten and lain dormant for thousands of years. With this awakened state comes the realization that we as humans are part of an inter-galactic family that is evolving along with the cosmos itself."

In *Unfolding Our Light* I explore the Oversouls further, adding crystals as well as entirely new information on the eighth, ninth and earth star chakras. The attunements presented here developed from communications with the Oversouls themselves. They seek to remind us of and to bring more depth to who we really are.

To understand an Oversoul we must first contemplate mandala forms. When we walk into a sacred place, be it a church, mosque, stone circle, synagogue or any building of spiritual importance we often sense a special presence. This is due to the awareness of the builders of such places and their ability to distill and use sacred geometry, proportions and harmonic principles in the design process, in order to enhance the energies that already existed there.

The fine details behind the patterns refer to the relationship between ourselves and our universe. The builders are seeking to expand and elevate our consciousness via the design to a higher spatial level of awareness. The intricate details of such places remind us of those principles and underlying patterns of creation that apparently exist within us and the universe itself.

These places serve to reflect back to us the sacred patterning of manifested creation. When we enter such places our aura feels attracted, senses the awareness behind these designs and can, if we are open to it, align accordingly. These same principles apply to the Oversoul temples and templates. Their visual manifestation as mandalas are purposeful. The intricate, never-ending and overlapping patterns within each temple are unique. Every fine detail stimulates our consciousness to remember aspects of our vastness; to reconnect with the awareness of our divine self.

Mandala is a Sanskrit word meaning circle. Nature expresses itself in many circular forms from shells, flowers, buds, to water bubbles, the list is endless. The circular theme varies throughout the world creating a multitude of sacred patterns. Many ancient traditions use mandalas to frame meditational, devotional and sacred ideas in a contained space. Mandalas focus not only us but what we have invoked. When we create one for ourselves, another or a group, we create protection, not from something outside of ourselves but from our own everyday distractions. Working with the mandalas in this way unlocks codes within our being and DNA.

These codes have been waiting for a particular moment in time which align with many ancient prophecies that point towards our collective initiation. I believe that grand alignment is happening right now and that many people are incarnate to witness and participate in it. A mandala creates a space for our consciousness to be transformed.

Using this book practically, we offer ourselves to be attuned and the crystal Oversouls for each attunement serve this purpose. Once activated through a mandala, they will saturate our being with their consciousness, and will help to elevate, attune and balance whatever needs it most.

When we invite the Oversouls into healing or meditation, these intricate energies and principles are brought into our physical reality and will adjust and expand it accordingly. We can, if we are open to it, participate consciously in the endlessly varied and dancing oneness of the universe. We can experience with our physical body the patterns of the stars, earth and the flows of creation surging, moving exquisitely through us.

In these attunements it is crystals that play a central role as transmitters and gateways for the energy of the new. Following a series of meditations within the Oversoul temples I understood that the Oversouls transmit themselves via a crystal or a crystals matrix. Within the Oversoul temples themselves are crystal guardians that reflect the Oversoul's awareness. These guardians are inter-connected with the mindset of the Oversoul.

They carry their mindset further, extending it into the consciousness of a crystal's matrix. When we then work with a crystal we are intrinsically linked directly to that crystal's Oversoul and vice versa. When we participate in the attunements in this book we are linking in through the crystals and Oversoul cards directly to the source of the temples and in doing so we draw those exquisite vibrations in towards ourselves, into the deeper consciousness of humanity. This is all part of a process whereby we have, on a soul level, agreed to participate in not only our own awakening but also humanity's.

***

Crystal beings have always had a strong relationship with humans. When we look at a crystal we might see beauty and order but if we also look further with our inner eye we may see beings who themselves have their own evolution and consciousness that is independent of ours. Crystals are physical manifestations and extended consciousness of an Oversoul on our plane of consciousness. A crystal is itself overseen by a Deva, an etheric form that distills its intelligence via the crystal.

A crystal is the bridge, the conduit for the power to travel into our world. When we direct our healing or intent through a crystal, it is amplifying the consciousness of an Oversoul and Deva directly into our aura. This sacred energy then circulates throughout our aura and chakra system, eventually filtering into our physical body. Through this action certain zones of our aura, depending on the crystal applied, can begin to expand to remember their vast potential.

This process encourages us to unfurl, to awaken, to open the door of perception that allow us to dream our life into being in a far wider perspective. For example, an understanding of working with Devas and an ancient healing power, anchored subtly in the matter around us.

Lemuria retreated into the ethers thousands of years ago. Having served its purpose, this great civilization did not need to be material. No longer supported by the energies of Lemuria, the great temples and the beings of stellar dimensions that also inhabited this world, we became less than we were. In Lemuria our chakra and aura system reflected a wider perspective of our consciousness. Our chakra centres of communication and sight were greatly enhanced, we were able to see, speak with and hear dimensions that have since become invisible.

Within these dimensions were many beings that we still refer to in myths and fables such as crystal beings, unicorns and elementals. As we learn to work with our eighth, ninth and earth star chakras and the corresponding levels of our auric field, we will start to see what was once invisible.

The beings that occupy these dimensions are returning to our conscious awareness and with this returns a sense of shared responsibility that we carry for these kingdoms. We once took a far stronger role in supporting the previously unseen kingdoms.

As we see, hear and communicate with them they become allies in our collective journey towards a new wholeness. This is all a part of our collective initiation. What had to become invisible will become, for some, visible.

How to use this book

Each chapter consists of an overview and a practical layout which involves particular crystals and mandalas involving crystal Oversoul cards.

There are 44 Oversoul cards, which have been arranged in such a way that all 44 are spread over all ten attunements. For each attunement in-depth information is provided on the auric layers, colours, sound and characteristics of its corresponding chakra. Each attunement and its corresponding mandala is aligned with a specific combination of crystals that is also explored.

Each chapter explores the attunements step by step, from the base to crown chakra. The book contains completely new material on the eighth, ninth and earth star chakra and their attunements. Together these attunements support an awakening of our vast potential.

Each of the following attunements is designed to be flexible, allowing for our expanded multi-dimensional awareness that knows what to do for our highest good. The way I understand working with the attunements presented here, is that the process will be relative to the amount of inner work you have previously put in and continue to do. You can work from the first attunement upwards or start with whichever one you feel drawn to.

I would recommend coming back to the information from time to time as attunements are ongoing exercises and will change each time we set out to begin them. The energy of an attunement follows divine intelligence in accordance with our free will.

You can use the information in this book in another way too. There are numerous crystals for each attunement that, if you are drawn to, can be meditated on. The final chapter of this book shows how to make essences for each attunement.

On the following pages there are some pictures that reflect different ways of creating the mandalas shown in this book, from group meditations to personal and Earth healing.

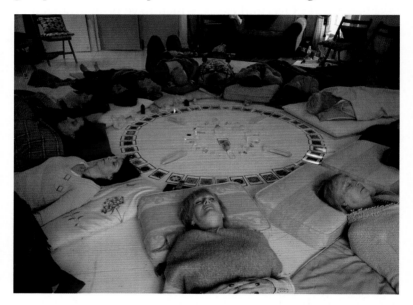

The above picture is taken from a workshop in 2012. During the day I created a mandala with all 44 of the crystal Oversoul cards. Once the cards were in place I added numerous crystals and then everyone else added any crystals of their own. I then guided the group into a meditation attunement.

This creates an extremely powerful group energy which greatly magnifies the attunement process. There are many variations for this exercise as each group will draw a unique response from the Oversouls depending on the needs of the group.

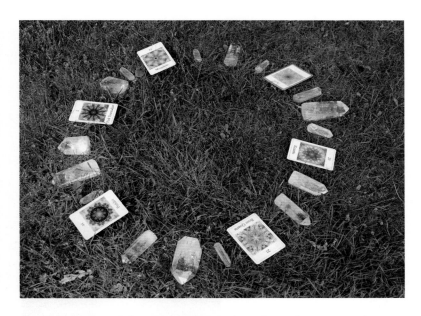

Simple mandalas with Oversoul cards and quartz points

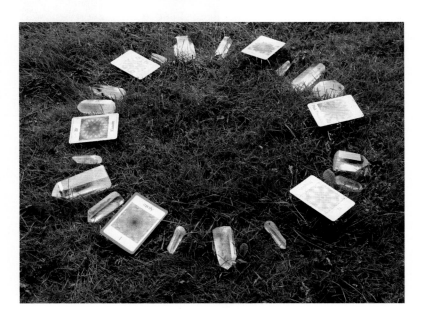

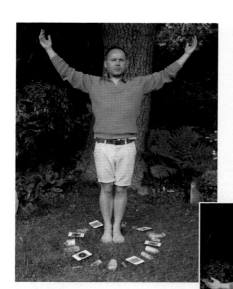

A mandala created for a standing meditation. Using various Crystal Oversoul cards as well as quartz points. This grid was made especially for an Earth healing ceremony in 2012 – drawing the energy into the Earth.

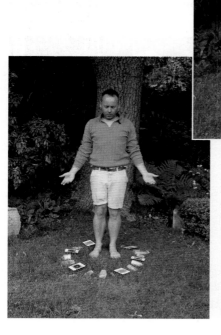

The First Attunement

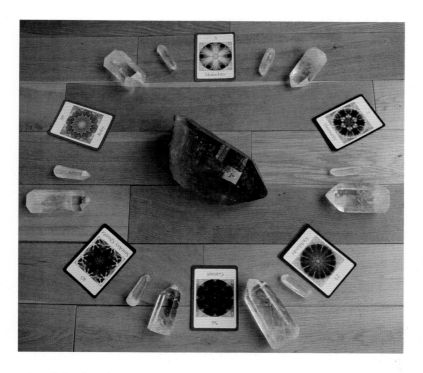

Mandala for the First Attunement: as long as all the Crystal Oversoul cards mentioned are used, feel free to add any or all of the crystals mentioned. In the above picture I have added a Smokey Quartz as well as many quartz points. If a crystal is added to your mandala, make sure you read what that particular crystal will bring into your attunement.

Crystals: Smokey Quartz, Red Garnet, Boji Stones, Chalcopyrite, Hematite, Brookite, Black Tourmaline, Ilvaite, Magnetite, Moldavite, Black Obsidian, Ruby, Shungite, Smokey Elestial Quartz, Fire Agate, Red Zincite, Malachite.

Crystal Oversoul cards: Malachite , Hematite, Moldavite, Garnet, Smokey Quartz, Ruby

Overview

Chakra Subject: Survival, boundaries, trust & security.

Body position of chakra: Base of spine, between anus and genitals.

Organs & glands: Affects heart rate, adrenal glands, muscles, feet, legs, coccyx, reproductive organs, colon, lower spine, sacrum, kidneys and bladder.

Tree of life position: Malkuth

Colour of chakra: Red

Musical Note: C

Seed syllable: Lam

Archangel: Sandolphon

Element: Earth

The first attunement has its primary focus on the etheric body and base chakra. The Crystal Oversoul temples of Malachite, Hematite, Moldavite, Garnet, Smokey Quartz and Ruby combine forces to activate, attune and strengthen the etheric body as well as the base chakra. If we also add any of the crystals; Smoky Quartz, Red Garnet, Boji Stones, Chalcopyrite, Hematite, Brookite, Black Tourmaline, Ilvaite, Magnetite, Moldavite, Black Obsidian, Ruby, Shungite, Smokey Elestial quartz, Fire Agate, Red Zincite and Malachite, we have the beginning of our journey.

Layout for the First Attunement

If you resonate with this attunement read the following writing first. Familiarize yourself with as much of the information as possible. You can do this process as many times as you like. Each time will be different because it affects another moment of your journey.

Decide if you are to lie within the mandala, sit or stand.

Lay the named crystal Oversoul cards in a mandala matching the position of your body.

Choose any of the mentioned crystals or all of them. All the ones you choose will be drawn into the energetic mixture. Another option is to decide different quantities of the same stone, for example six Malachite. Be creative and trust your intuition. Lay these crystals within the Oversoul mandala.

Once your mandala is laid out lay or stand inside the mandala. The crystal Oversoul cards provide a gateway for the energy necessary to protect, open and offer the created space for the attunement. Relax, resting with the support of the crystal consciousness and its innate ability to transport you to the level and frequency that is correct for you. There is nothing you need to direct. The more you relax and allow, the deeper the process can become.

It is difficult to say for how long the process lasts as this work has a time all of its own. An obvious drop in energy can be felt when the process is complete.

First Auric Layer

Etheric —- *Element:* Earth

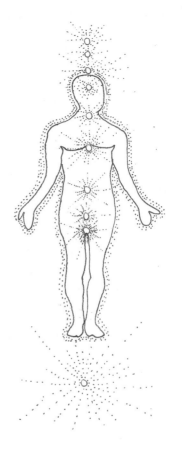

Each layer of our aura, although individual, is part of the intelligent web of life that serves our divinity.

As we move, extending away from the physical body, we encounter the etheric layer, which radiates out from the physical body by a couple of inches and surrounds it entirely. It envelopes and mirrors the body's shape and size and has a luminous blue shine.

Through this body weave the chakras, meridians and chi lifeforce carry energy down from less dense levels into the physical body. If this body is healthy it will radiate vitality. What determines the health and vitality of this part of our aura is our attitude to health, exercise and nutrition. We also need to take into account our genetic makeup.

At this level of our being we can effect its vitality by exercising, eating well and treating ourselves with respect. If we neglect this body we can experience loss of vitality, inertia and lack of will power. At this level the more we put in the more we get out.

Each layer of the aura carries sound-waves. The etheric body, again depending on our health, holds a higher pitch than the physical body. People who care for their health will have not only a vibrant blue light emanating from this level but will also emit vibrant sounds. If we are blocked on this level the sounds will be dull and discordant.

If we are carrying denser energy on other layers of our aura this can in time start to impact upon the etheric body. It is like a weight starts to build up and, if left unaddressed, will push down on the etheric body and thus the physical body. The etheric is very much an interface between the physical body and all of the other subtle bodies of the aura. It is responsible for the transfer of life energy or vitality from the universal energy field to the physical body.

I look at this layer like a reflection of all the glands, organs and parts of the physical body, an x ray of the insides of a person on the outside. This image gives an indication of the energetic condition of a person for each organ, gland and part of the body. If healthy, it will be illuminated with life-force, if under nourished it will look dull, tired and lifeless.

The first attunement process strengthens this body offering a new template of health and vitality. This can be a powerful attunement for those experiencing lack in their lives.

First Chakra ~ Base

The first attunement opens us to understanding that it is better to flow with life's experiences, not to stagnate but to move forwards with trust in the process. The physical plane is one of constant movement and change. Our human personalities are vehicles for the expression on this plane and in this lifetime and will dissolve upon our death.

Learning to be in our body, to enjoy its pleasures and not to get attached to it is one of the keys to health.

No chakra can stand on its own, all of the chakras interact and relate with each other.

This attunement opens our base chakra to receiving more pranic energy. This is crucial as it functions as the foundation, which enables us to stand firmly on the soil of the earth.

When our base chakra is healthy and clear we know we can take positive steps to achieve our goals, we believe in our own ability to create and shape reality. We feel connected to humanity and know that life and being a part of this world is a divine gift and blessing. We experience that heaven is here, expressing itself through us. The base chakra is the furthest away from the crown and this is the most primal of all our chakras.

Without the base chakra balanced our consciousness and personality will not have much spare time for the higher ideals of the other chakras. You will see, as we go through each chakra, that they each have their place in the scheme of things and each one interacts with the others. If our personality is fretting about survival and security issues then this chakra is going to be draining energy and awareness from the other chakras.

The first three to four years of our childhood will set the tone for the base chakra, as this is a crucial stage in our development. If we had warm, supportive early years, felt nurtured, safe and loved then this chakra will often not be an issue. If we experienced upheaval, distress, unclear boundaries and abandonment up to this age, then the tone will be set very differently and until this chakra is balanced life will simply not go to plan.

People who have difficult first three to four years will often show symptoms of distrust, depression and either hidden anger or sudden outbursts of anger. They will often feel that in order to stand on their own feet they need to work obsessively as though that will bring the peace they so desire, or become dependent on others for their sense of identity and security, all with an overriding need for outside approval. This is, often enough, set to fail though as that is not the way the universe works. By learning from and balancing the base chakra, the obsessive focus on survival, tension and control eases and life takes on a sweeter note.

This means dealing more consciously with the reality of one's presence in the world, with the earth plane issues such as stability, trust, boundaries, money, responsibility, letting go and discernment. Some of the signs that the base chakra is not functioning to its fullest expression are inertia, an inability to take action, loss of feeling and spacyness.

This attunement offers strength by clearing the pathways around the base chakra of discordant energies of stress, anxiety and fear. Through this attunement we are offered ways of attaining a new attitude towards survival issues. The base chakra, rather than contracting through fear or anxiety, expands, is invited to become open and receptive to new potential and solutions.

The Oversouls for the First Attunement

There are six Oversouls aligned to this attunement. Interestingly a cube, representing the Earth element, has six faces. Each of the six Oversouls is powerful in its own right – they start to build the most incredible energy. Each of these Oversouls connects to the base chakra by helping to restore this sacred gateway of our body to its full potential, on the one hand and, on the other hand individually or collectively to strengthen our boundaries.

Together the six Oversouls create a consciousness in form of a cube that extends into our etheric body, symbolising a strengthened and addressed Earth chakra.

Malachite has many important healing qualities. It can help us learn to trust the earth and the cycles of creation. Through the vibration of this stone we face life and feel that we can handle our experience on the physical plane.

Malachite's growth can remind us of more flexible ways of integrating structure and discipline, helping us understand these functions that are vital to carry out projects.

Working with Malachite helps us realize that we have the right to take our space in the world. It is a powerful healing ally helping us to understand control issues. Its message is 'trust yourself and life – leave room for the unknown and unexpected'. The Malachite Oversoul plays an important role in our development. When used for healing or meditation this Oversoul can illuminate our journey through human history. Our sense of compassion towards ourself is enhanced as we come to recognize that through the eyes of the universe we are unique. The gifts we have brought to humanity's growth although not always recognized, has been important.

Malachite has a special role within the framework of this attunement as it encourages us to take our space in the world. Within its temple structure our ancient glyphs activate every time we connect with this Oversoul. Our etheric body and base chakra become illuminated through any interaction we have with the Malachite Oversoul. We expand rather than contract. This recalibrates both the etheric and base chakra to a new frequency that is trusting as well as open.

Hematite helps us ground ourselves by encouraging and maintaining boundaries. By working with this crystal a person's energy radiance becomes strong and healthy. This can lead to the energy field deflecting any external influences that would otherwise deplete a person's life force. Hematite helps one stay clear and vibrant by establishing a healthy relationship with the earth plane.

In some cultures and lifetimes there has been a tradition of neglecting the human body, with the deceptive promise to become more spiritual. Hematite is a great crystal companion for people who feel that they have not been able to honour their body and experience a division between body and soul. When we apply this Oversoul's energy to the base chakra we open the meridian lines from the base chakra right down into the earth. We can start to feel not only a connection to the earth but also that we belong and are wanted.

Hematite has a unique place in the attunement process as it assists people who feel that they don't want to be incarnate. The energy matrix of this Oversoul offers us a feeling of safety, one that embraces change and uncertainty. Helping us find peace with the earth and our body, through accepting that change, is beautiful.

There are times in most peoples' lives where a leap of faith is called for. **Moldavite** is the perfect crystal companion during such times. Its energy encourages flexibility, spontaneity and dexterity. With this stone's energy by our side we know we can achieve our goals. We take the necessary actions, certain that the right set of opportunities are at hand. We are able to follow our inner guidance as we have cultivated the ability to listen to the signs from an intuitive level. We have examined our motives and desires and know that what we are creating is in our best interest: it will bring us pleasure.

There are endless possibilities with Moldavite as it encourages us to expand our horizons and open our mind to new experiences. If we apply this energy to the base chakra we can support an expansion of this chakra's possibilities.

In the Moldavite Oversoul temple walls are many ancient star codes that trigger memories. These memories serve to quicken the energy of the etheric body by clearing discordant patterns that are inhibiting this layer of our being.

Garnet reminds us that within our body and soul dwells the same spark of creation that gave birth to worlds within worlds. We carry the fire of endless possibilities and creativity in our being. Our work on earth is to encourage and enliven this spark within and make the world a better place for us being in it. This crystal emanates a dynamic and inventive energy we can draw upon when we find it a struggle to relate to ourselves or the world.

There comes a quickening, a speeding of personal evolution with Garnet. Meditating with this stone will clear any patterns that are inhibiting or restricting the expression of the divine spark in the base of the spine. Garnet helps us find the courage to make any changes we need to make our life express itself with the highest of light.

Smokey Quartz is a master crystal, helping us to ground inner experiences into a workable reality. It reminds us to make proper use of our foundation and personality. If we are out of sync with the requirements of the earth plane, then this is the stone to meditate with. Smokey quartz carries the warm browns and black tones of the Earth and we can be open to learn from this master.

If you desire to manifest a dream into reality and it is running against the flow of society or is ahead of its time, then Smokey quartz will be the perfect companion. Through the vibrational structure of Smoky quartz we can learn how the game of life works and understand how our dream will fit in.

The Smokey quartz Oversoul is a master of patience. Seek its wise counsel if you find that you are getting frustrated with trying to make things happen. This wise being attunes us to qualities of diligence, steadfastness and perseverance.

The deeply warming qualities of **Ruby** activate our life force and primal powers located deep within the base chakra. This gives us the power to act upon our intuition and take the necessary steps to making things happen. Ruby has a long association with the qualities of leadership and power because its energy stimulates activity and action, thus decision making. Ruby helps to cut through inertia and depression forging the way ahead into possibilities. Ruby is overseen by the Lords of Karma and if used wisely, will help us to push through the cloudy vision of karmic entanglements. Ruby encourages us ultimately to cultivate a consciousness of service.

The Ruby Oversoul, through the first attunement, clears karmic memory from the etheric body as well as the base chakra. This memory can have had many functions that have served our being until now. Through this attunement we have the opportunity, with the support of the Lords of Karma, to be clear.

The Crystals for the First Attunement

All of these crystals fit within the framework of the first attunement. You could choose all from the list and place them in your circle. Alternatively choose one crystal that appeals to you, build a mandala and place the crystal in the centre. Or choose a few from the list that appeal, placing them throughout the circle. There are no rules so be creative and trust yourself.

Smokey Quartz is perfectly positioned to assist us in balancing the base chakra. Through its dark smokey tones this chakra is aligned to feelings of security and balance on the earth plane. The energies of this crystal ask us to learn to support ourselves by being kinder and more patient. Many beings carry past life memories of hardship and difficulty with the earth and physical bodies. Smokey Quartz can illuminate these patterns and if we desire will assist us in letting them go.

Through this act of release we can come to experience the earth and our body as a place of safety and beauty. This beautiful crystal is perfectly aligned to assist with the first attunement, asking us to relax, to begin to experience the Earth as a place that nurtures our life-force and creativity.

Red Garnet asks us to meditate on and to experience the divine spark that flows and surges within the deeper layers of our body. We may carry karmic memories within the base of our spine and base chakra, that have taught us to neglect our life force, to remain less than we are and powerless. If we desire, Red Garnet, within the context of this attunement, will support us in releasing any patterns of powerlessness. It does this by supporting our attention on this subject with our willingness to release the past, to set ourselves free. Through this action we create the space within our body for the new to materialize.

Boji Stones offer a sense of reverence, honour and humility towards our physical existence. Boji Stones as healing companions, offer us balance and wholeness through an alchemical union of our inner masculine and feminine energies. Through working with these stones, the base chakra comes to understand that it is time to release itself from identifying with archetypes of separate forces; that once we balance and bring our male and female forces together we experience wholeness within ourselves. The base chakra can then operate from a higher vibration and release the conflict of polarisation.

Chalcopyrite is a wonderful healing ally helping us through periods of inertia and apathy. It is especially powerful when used in this attunement because of its emphasis on balancing the base chakra as well as the etheric body.

Hematite is a potent healer of the base chakra through its unique ability that encourages us to strengthen our boundaries. Through its powers we are more than able to know what is the right vibration for us and our needs. We learn to eliminate the need to be held back or put down by others. The etheric body in particular is reminded that it is there to protect and store our essence. Within the framework of the first attunement this crystal serves to remind us that we are powerful beings of light and matter, that we are capable of supporting our needs on the Earth. Hematite has a deeply healing presence, encouraging us to enjoy our physical body within the world of form and matter.

Brookite has a very high and unique vibration. It assists in the awakening of ancient energies lain dormant in our base chakra for many lifetimes, awaiting this current age of light. Through its awakening and activation of deeper currents within the base chakra we come into a powerful stage of our awakening. We imbue the base with very strong currents of energy that are important to complete the tasks in this lifetime. Through our interaction with this stone we learn how to rejuvenate our life force by allowing ancient activation codes to begin to unfurl. Brookite's deep healing rays penetrate the base chakra, illuminating any apathy that is holding us back from fully embracing life.

Black Tourmaline is an important ally in our awakening journey as its energy assists us to draw out of our aura excessive negative and harmful toxic energy. For some people these energies have been carried around in their astral bodies from many lifetimes and can impede the person's expansion. If we are carrying toxic vibrations in our astral bodies the base chakra can become burdened and unable to function. Its ability to process and eliminate can be greatly affected. Black tourmaline is a master mineral in its clarity and determination to help us become free of toxins and live a fully richer life.

Ilvaite is a great assistant in these times as it helps us if we need to feel the support of the universe. If we carry an attitude of resentment towards the world then Ilvaite is a powerful healing crystal. Discovering our attitude towards something can be a powerful force for change. With the right attitude we can create miracles in our lives. Ilvaite seeks to remind us that the universe will support us with each step we take but we must first of all allow ourselves to trust. We are often asked to trust in forces we cannot see or hear. The first attunement in conjunction with Ilvaite seeks to address this, allowing us to remain true to our light and open to guidance.

Magnetite has a unique role to play in our development. Magnetite can help us stay focused and grounded on what is in this moment. This can have a powerful impact on our well-being as once we are here, in the moment, we can consider many more possibilities. Our base chakra, although spinning at a slower rate than the other chakras, can become overstimulated when we are not present to the moment. Magnetite encourages us to breathe into the safety of present moment awareness.

Moldavite is one of the most important crystals for this age of light. Moldavite has an accelerated frequency that assists us in letting go of karmic residue that serves no purpose in this lifetime. The base chakra is aligned and restored to our original essence, released from any vows or any karmic imprints that are designed to keep us small.

During the first attunement Moldavite illuminates the ancient flame that resides within our base chakra. Once active in the base chakra this flame then illuminates the etheric body. This flame is designed to be activated during important points in human acceleration. Such a time is at hand and Moldavite is aware of us and awaits permission to activate. Moldavite will, upon activation of this flame, assist in bringing all we need to complete our journey.

Black Obsidian is perfectly suited to settle certain traits within our being. When we work with this stone we can start to face any hurdles we have placed within our own way. These hurdles may be beliefs that have shaped who we are or attitudes that are imprisoning our life force. This is one of the most powerful of all the crystals as it mirrors back to us exactly what it is we are sending out into the world. Black Obsidian is like the astrological planet Pluto whose role is to illuminate and free us only from that which does not serve us. Black Obsidian can lead us towards deep healing.

Ruby is perfectly aligned to assist us in illuminating the fire within our base chakra. If we have difficulties in holding firm to our values or integrity then Ruby will step forward to support us. Our Soul pours out its light through our physical heart and our eyes. Ruby assists us in coming to know this light and letting it guide and support us through our journey of life. Through the attunement process we can begin to learn from our Soul's light, allowing it to guide and nourish us.

Shungite has a unique role to play in the healing of the base chakra. It comes into its own when there is a build-up of emotional debris within the base chakra. Shungite's penetrating rays can illuminate and help transmute discordant patterns that are impeding health and well- being. These patterns, once released from the base, are also released from any hold they have on the etheric body.

Through the first attunement we are supported in letting go of any addiction to the past that we may be identifying with. Shungite within the context of this attunement, seeks to help us understand parts of ourselves that cling to the past even if that past no longer serves us.

Smokey Elestial Quartz is a master crystal having a special relationship within the first attunement, as it reconnects our consciousness to Devic and Angelic fields of light. Through this attunement we have the opportunity to align ourselves with missing elements of our vaster being. The forces of Devic and Angelic light expand our awareness, remind us of the energies that build and maintain creation. When we come into contact with this energy we are reminded, on a cellular level, that as human beings we play an important part in the co-creation of many other kingdoms. This includes elemental forms.

When we recognize the importance of these other kingdoms and their maintenance of the web of creation we become more than humans just being alive. We can start to step forward as the vast multi-dimensional beings that we are.

Fire Agate can play an important role in our journey to union. We carry within us the seeds of endless possibilities and if we forget this can lose our passion for life. Fire Agate reminds the core memory within the base chakra of its unlimited potential to create. Through this we can come to know, on a deep level of our being, that we ourselves are creativity in action. The first attunement restores membranes deep within the base chakra. This can have the effect of helping this centre be able to draw in more energy from the cosmos, enabling this chakra to operate more fully and take its role in supporting the influx of energy that this attunement creates.

Red Zincite supports us by helping us manifest and ground our ideas into physical reality. It asks us to take our imagination and dreams seriously, to see that these dreams are rising from the depths of our consciousness and that they mater. If you have a habit of procrastinating or thinking your dream is unreachable then this crystal is your guide for this attunement or for further meditation.

Malachite is a powerful reminder that we are meant to take our space within the world. We matter in the eyes of the universe. Through working with this stone the base chakra learns to relax and not hold on too tightly. This can have the healing effect of encouraging our minds and heart to let go, feeling supported by the universe.

The Second Attunement

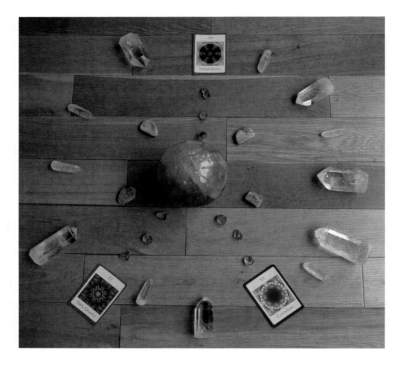

Mandala for the Second Attunement: as long as all the Crystal Oversoul cards mentioned are used, feel free to add any or all of the crystals mentioned. In the above picture I have added a Honey calcite and four Moonstones as well as many quartz points. If a crystal is added to your mandala, make sure you read what that particular crystal will bring into your attunement.

Crystals: Fairy quartz, Rutilated Quartz, Orange Zincite, Tantric twin, Honey Calcite, Isis crystal, Carnelian Creedite, Moonstone, Opal.

Crystal Oversoul cards: Moonstone, Carnelian, Fairy Quartz.

Overview

Chakra Subject: Creativity & passion.

Body position: Genitals, lower back.

Organs & glands: Ovaries, testicles, kidneys, skin.

Tree of life position: Yesod

Colour: Orange

Musical Note: D

Seed syllable: Vam

Archangel: Gabriel

Element: Water

The second attunement has its primary focus on the emotional body and sacral chakra. The Crystal Oversoul temples of Moonstone, Carnelian and Fairy Quartz combine forces to activate, attune and strengthen the emotional body as well as the sacral chakra. If we also add any of the crystals (Fairy quartz, Rutilated Quartz, Orange Zincite, Tantric twin, Honey Calcite, Isis crystal, Carnelian, Harlequin quartz, Creedite, Moonstone and Opal), they can add some subtle aspects to our attunement.

Layout for the Second Attunement

If you resonate with this attunement read the following writing first. Familiarize yourself with as much of the information as possible. You can do this process as many times as you like. Each time will be different because it affects another moment of your journey.

Decide if you are to lie within the mandala, sit or stand.

Lay the named crystal Oversoul cards in a mandala matching the position of your body.

Choose any of the mentioned crystals or all of them. All the ones you choose will be drawn into the energetic mixture. Another option is to decide different quantities of the same stone, for example, twelve Moonstone. Be creative and trust your intuition. Lay these crystals within the Oversoul mandala.

Once your mandala is laid out lay or stand inside the mandala. The crystal Oversoul cards provide a gateway for the energy necessary to protect, open and offer the created space for the attunement. Relax, resting with the support of the crystal consciousness and its innate ability to transport you to the level and frequency that is correct for you. There is nothing you need to direct.

The more you relax and allow, the deeper the process can become.

It is difficult to say for how long the process lasts as this work has a time all of its own. An obvious drop in energy can be felt when the process is complete.

Second Auric Layer

Emotional — *Element:* Water

Moving on to the next layer of the auric field we extend our auric awareness further to meet the emotional or feeling body. The second attunement is associated with our feelings and emotional well-being.

How we perceive colours of this body will be determined by our feelings for ourselves and others. If we are positive, happy, healthy, content and present with our feelings then this body will reflect itself through a myriad of vibrant colours. These

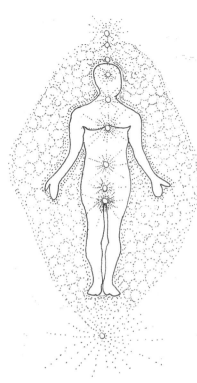

colours can be very attractive and pleasant to observe.

If on the other hand we are negative, resentful, unhappy, discontent, stuck or unable to express or feel our feelings then this will also be reflected through colours. These can take the form of dark patches that might look and feel unpleasant. This energy can clog and inhibit our life force from travelling freely though our bodies of light.

However the aura of this level reflects and mirrors how we feel, without any judgement.

The myriad of colour expressions on this layer can change moment by moment. If we are feeling stuck and experience a breakthrough the emotional body will reflect this immediately.

In my observation we are born with various signature colours on the emotional level. These colours are determined by previous lives and our parental/family choice in this lifetime. The vibrancy of our birth colours changes depending on the decisions we already make as children. If we accept the family patterns and leave them unchallenged our aura will remain essentially unchanged.

If on the other hand we change our attitude to our early family imprints we can change the vibrancy and colours associated to this layer. I have seen people change their entire colour patterning on this level through putting their inner work into practice. Where there were dark unexpressed pockets in their feeling body there are now free spaces, open for new ideas and feelings to be born into.

The emotional value of the colours we are transmitting on this level will strongly influence what we attract towards ourselves in life. On this level like attracts like. At birth our emotional body develops a strong bond primarily with a mothering energy. This can be with either parent or both depending on their energy. This body, with an affirmative support, stays connected with our parents until our teenage years.

From these years onwards we start to develop away from our parents protective field, needing to begin the process of experiencing life on our own feet. If this process is stifled, the emotional body will reflect frustration and create all sorts of issues. Thus the formative years will govern the overall well-being of the emotional body and its ability to reflect and support healthy choices as an adult. By no means does that indicate that we experience a dysfunctional upbringing, the process will present more challenges. Our parents inhibit this process by keeping us too close, and not letting us start to leave their influence can cause compulsion, helplessness and neediness to arise.

We may not know how to look after ourselves later in life, be able to handle finances, relationships or simply make mistakes while finding our own way in the world.

If we have an upbringing within a same sex or a single parent framework the aura develops the same way. A child's aura will interconnect with the aura of a primary person seeking to be nurtured in a mothering way.

The emotional body makes a gentle vibrant humming that matches the colours dancing around a person's field. One may hear a person humming or quietly singing, not aware that they are doing so. Or they may listen to music that reflects this mood.

The second attunement carries an enormous healing potential on the level of what we have learnt to feel. If we are ready to open, develop and learn from our feelings, the emotional body will attract experiences that reflect these changes. Thus, this attunement serves to elevate and recalibrate the emotional body patterns that underline our reality like an invisible matrix.

Second Chakra ~ Sacral

The sacral chakra swirls just over our reproductive organs. It rules our feelings which flow like water, our body, emotions, sexual drive, creativity, orientation and subconscious responses to events. The sacral chakra is the home of our personal dreams and gestation, where the new is born and nurtured. It is the place where we can take care of ourselves, learn to honour the nuances of our inner needs, trust and protect our inner dreams. The water element gives movement and fluidity to all the other chakras, and without this mix there would be no life force.

The signal that the sacral chakra is not receiving enough pranic energy or has been damaged can be found on many levels of a person. On the level of the physical body, difficulties can express themselves through impotence, difficulties around the testicles, kidneys, skin and ovaries.

Sexual abuse has an immense impact on the sacral chakra and the emotional body, more than any other area. When we lose faith in another through a loss of trust this centre can become damaged and closes, possibly resulting in feelings of coldness and a strong sense of isolation in a person.

The past will need to come to the surface to be released. When working with clients be mindful of the possible reality that ancient or recent memories can surface, make sure you can understand and address these memories and be of help to the client to process the past and incorporate them into an understandable reality.

The signal that this centre is not functioning healthily is getting stuck in the past, unable to move beyond past experiences, impotence, addictions, frigidity, fear, sexual abuse, emotional abuse. This centre also deals with how we digest on physical and emotional level; events that shock us greatly affect this place. When the second attunement is taken the sacral is encouraged to open and flow. We can trust our feelings to act as guidance for what is right for us, we strengthen our trust in people and the world.

The sacral chakra is the source of our desire to create. This manifests in society as male and female couples that choose to give birth to children, but creativity is not just about giving birth to physical children. We can give birth to creative ideas and projects, just as important as children. We can co-create whatever we desire to and we are all living art forms, our lives are our creative pursuits. Through the second attunement we are able to nurture creativity in ourselves and others, seeing that the birth and protection of ideas hold the key to life itself.

The Oversouls for the Second Attunement

There are three Oversouls aligned to this attunement. Interestingly the number 3 in numerology supports this figure. Number 3 represents creativity, inspiration and the arts – as well as the ability to overcome adversity. The second attunement is very aligned to these subjects. The Moonstone, Carnelian and Fairy quartz Oversouls on their own are deeply healing and nurturing. When we put them together for this attunement we are aligned emotionally in ways that serves, heals and thus uplift our spirits.

The Moonstone Oversoul balances the sacral chakra that oversees the water element of the body. When the water element of the body is flowing, the etheric body is more open and relaxed. All human beings have active and receptive sides to their nature, represented by fire (active) and water (receptive). This alchemical relationship between fire and water is the creative mixture that shapes our life. In order to successfully create reality we must have a balanced relationship with both sides. Moonstone draws us towards the waters of our receptive, open nature. Here we learn the qualities of listening, trusting, eliminating, flowing with the unknown and being patient. These qualities will be more necessary for us as we learn to navigate the unknown.

The Moonstone Oversoul serves as a guide as we travel deeper into the unknown. This beautiful Oversoul guards our energy during times of uncertainty for humans and humanity as a whole. As we move further into a new matrix or new earth we are faced with choices that humanity has not needed to make before. Lean into this Oversoul's light to feel the knowingness that all is going to plan.

The Carnelian Oversoul is a being of great creativity and flexibility. This potent ally stimulates and balances the sacral chakra and can bring renewed vitality and enhance creative pleasure. Our natural curiosity is aroused through working with this crystal, thus our minds and hearts are directed to finding solutions and opportunities. This is the crystal to have around if you are experiencing upheaval or great changes in your life. Its vibration is a tonic for strained nerves and helps to settle fears. With this stone by your side change becomes something to be excited about, an opportunity for the new to flow into your life. The future is positive and only the best will happen.

The Carnelian Oversoul helps to return our consciousness to peace. The attunement aligns the emotional body and sacral chakra in ways that have not been available to us before.

The Fairy Quartz Oversoul is here to remind us to pay attention to the small details, to learn to play and experience the magic of creation. Fairy quartz helps reconnect to one's inner child and is a special aid for working on abandonment issues. This crystal supports our journey by encouraging us to trust, to allow our guard to come down so that we can reconnect and feel the warmth of our heart.

The Fairy Quartz Oversoul connects us to elemental kingdoms that require our deepest respect. These kingdoms are important in healing, serving to remind us that we need to respect other forms of life and co-create with them in mind.

The Crystals for the Second Attunement

All of these crystals fit within the framework of the second attunement. You could choose all from the list and place them in your circle. Alternatively choose one crystal that appeals to you, build a mandala and place the crystal in the centre. Or choose a few from the list that appeal, placing them throughout the circle. There are no rules so be creative and trust yourself.

Fairy Quartz plays a unique role in our healing journey. Fairy energy is secretive, wild & mysterious, opening us to our adventurous nature which yearns to explore what the world has to offer. During the second attunement Fairy quartz aligns the sacral chakra to a new flow of experiences, reminding us to pay attention to the small details, to learn to play and experience the magic of creation.

Rutilated Quartz assists in getting any stagnant or trapped energy in the sacral chakra moving. When we encounter this crystal the rutile needles within the quartz quicken the energy currents that flow through this chakra. This has the effect of illuminating any blockages and releasing them.

During the second attunement we can learn to experience clarity and transformation that may have been hidden due to the blockage. Rutilated Quartz can also help us come to terms with our past, to clear the subconscious of fears and anxieties and reflect positive images of ourselves and life.

Orange Zincite is suited to opening us to the flow of new energies and ideas. If we have become stagnant or closed off to the new this crystal encourages us to take a deep breath and let go. When used in conjunction with the second attunement Orange Zincite brings an air of excitement to our healing journey, quickening our openness for change.

Tantric Twin Quartz are two separate crystal points sharing a common base. These rare crystals help to balance our male and female polarities bringing us into an alchemical union with our deeper self. Through this crystal we can come to know that we need seek no other to complete us. This does not mean we do not need others to be with and enjoy the company of, on the contrary it means that we can be with others without needing to draw from them what we are lacking. This can make for a whole new pattern of love and relationships. During the second attunement this sacred crystal assists us in moving onto a whole new matrix of experience, one where we honour ourselves as the source of what we are seeking.

Honey Calcite is here is help us stay aligned whilst experiencing changes on the outer reality of life. It gently reminds us to keep allowing and believing that the changes have arisen from ourselves, deep within our being. This honey coloured crystal supports us in knowing that we are co-creators of our life. From this knowing arises a strong faith in our own power to shape our life.

Isis Crystals are a variety of quartz that exhibit a five sided face on one side of the main apex. It is linked to the Goddess Isis through its association with the Isis and Osiris archetypes. The Goddess Isis overcame seemingly insurmountable adversity to search for and piece together the body of Osiris so that he could ascend. This crystal can teach us much about the qualities of perseverance, self-healing and overcoming great odds. When we apply this crystal in the second attunement, we are assisted in our healing through the emergence of many ancient, forgotten fragments of our being. We are reminded of the missing pieces of our vastness that remained hidden from view. Once drawn back in to our attention, what was hidden becomes visible. Through this we realize that these fragments are missing pieces of the garment of light that together complete our light-body.

Carnelian is a good stone for those who feel that they have something creative to bring to the world, but feel inhibited by lack of direction. It can bring courage of conviction, a positive self-image and the realization that we are here to birth the new into our lives. We experience that we each have a unique gift to bring to this world. Carnelian's orange vibration is sensed by the soul plane of our being. It can be called upon to release grief or sadness from the subconscious levels. If there have been lives of pain, hardship or torture, these memories can reside deeply in the subconscious. When we apply Carnelian in the second attunement we encourage the grief, over time, to surface and re-lease.

Through this letting go, we can become open for new energies to be received by our subconscious, especially the qualities of joy. Through Carnelian we can access the sea of joy and learn to experience with our whole body the joy of being part of the world.

Creedite has a light joyous quality, firstly through the colour it exhibits and secondly its powerful presence. It carries very high levels of light that raises everything in its vicinity to a higher plane of awareness. When applied within the context of the second attunement, Creedite recalibrates our sacral chakra in such a way that we realize how important it is to bring our dreams into manifestation. If we find creating and living our dreams a challenge it can be that we are carrying belief patterns that are restricting our path. Creedite assists us in exploring what it is that we believe to be true and through inner work, releasing these beliefs if they do not serve us. We carry these dreams like seeds in the DNA of our soul. We are in a time that will support the germination of these seeds coming into reality.

Moonstone gets is sheen through the reflection of light from the layers of its internal structure. It is perfectly placed to assist in the second attunement. During this process we are reminded that we are deep flowing beings that are subject to powerful inner forces. These forces ask us to trust ourselves, to dive deep, to swim in the currents of our being. If we are open to it, this journey opens an allowance on our part for the past to be released. That which we are holding on to can begin to relax.

The sacral chakra is the gateway to our feelings, subconscious and deeper drives. Through this attunement, with the assistance of Moonstone, we become flexible to change and are able to flow with the wisdom of our being.

Opal (clear, white or water opals) are divine mirrors illuminating what it is we are projecting into the world. Opal asks us to look at ourselves with clarity and reflection. If we seek to blame the world or another person for our experience, this stone will remind us that it is our own attitude that creates our experiences. Until we take responsibility for our own energy emanation we will never find peace.

The Third Attunement

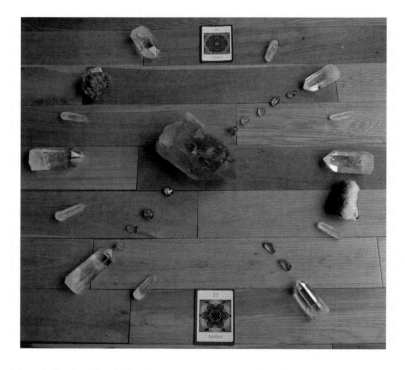

Mandala for the Third Attunement: as long as all the Crystal Oversoul cards mentioned are used, feel free to add any or all of the crystals mentioned. In the above picture I have added a Citrine point, Citrine clusters, Ambers as well as many quartz points. If a crystal is added to your mandala, make sure you read what that particular crystal will bring into your attunement.

Crystals: Lemurian Golden Healer, Citrine, Gold Tektite, Amblygonite, Faden quartz, Amber and Stellar Beam calcite

Crystal Oversoul cards: Amber, Citrine

Overview

Chakra Subject: Personal power.

Body position: Stomach.

Organs & glands: Stomach, digestion, gallbladder, liver, nervous system, pancreas, adrenals.

Tree position: Lower arc of Tiphareth.

Colour: Yellow

Musical Note: E

Seed syllable: Ram

Archangel: Michael

Element: Fire

The third attunement has its primary focus on the mental body and solar plexus chakra. The Crystal Oversoul temples of Amber and Citrine combine forces to activate, attune and initiate this layer of the aura as well as this chakra. If we also add any of the crystals; Lemurian Golden Healer, Citrine, Gold Tektite, Amblygonite, Faden quartz, Amber and Stellar Beam Calcite we can focus on some subtle aspects concerning the mental body and solar plexus chakra.

Layout for the Third Attunement

If you resonate with this attunement read the following writing first. Familiarize yourself with as much of the information as possible. You can do this process as many times as you are like. Each time will be different because it affects another moment of your journey.

Decide if you are to lie within the mandala, sit or stand.

Lay the named crystal Oversoul cards in a mandala matching the position of your body.

Choose any of the mentioned crystals or all of them. All the ones you choose will be drawn into the energetic mixture. Another option is to decide different quantities of the same stone, for example, four Citrine. Be creative and trust your intuition. Lay these crystals within the Oversoul mandala.

Once your mandala is laid out, lay or stand inside the mandala. The crystal Oversoul cards provide a gateway for the energy necessary to protect, open and offer the created space for the attunement. Relax, resting with the support of the crystal consciousness and its innate ability to transport you to the level and frequency that is correct for you. There is nothing you need to direct. The more you relax and allow, the deeper the process can become.

It is difficult to say for how long the process lasts as this work has a time all of its own. An obvious drop in energy can be felt when the process is complete.

Third Auric Layer

Mental – *Element:* Fire

As we extend our awareness further we meet the mental body. It is located above the emotional layer again surrounding the entire body. It governs our intellect as well as our intuition. When it is vibrant these two forces work together reflecting a vivid pale yellow colouring. Our intellectual clarity and agility is being mirrored on this level. When vivid in colour we have a strong sense of our own ideas and thoughts, being able to express these into the world. When this body works alongside the emotional feeling body we have a powerful developed connection between our feelings as well as our rational mind. We feel that

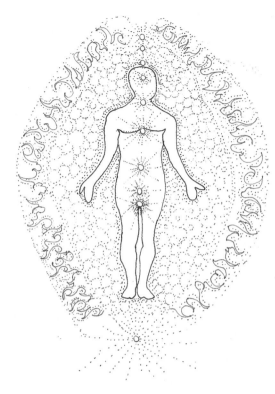

the two forces can work well, without the need to over develop one or the other.

If on the other hand we neglect this layer we may find that our thought processes are underdeveloped and we will have difficulty in making our ideas come into manifestation.

The mental body then becomes cloudy, muddled and unable to connect ideas or intuition into a cohesive picture.

We may also overstrengthen this layer if we are inhibited on an emotional level, hoping that through developing our mental body via our intellect we will not need to feel. This attitude creates a strong mental body that, although powerful, cannot act alone. There will come a time when the disowned emotions will seek a way to be heard.

Through this field of our aura we develop our impressions and attitude to life. If we remain negative this layer will remain close to the body getting more and more stagnant in its expression. The term having a closed mind has a powerful resonance with the mental body. If we limit the luminosity of this body through shutting ourselves off to new ideas, ways of thinking or ways of seeing then we in effect shut off the flow of fresh energy into this body. This can have the effect of closing this body down, becoming rigid and closed.

When we work within this body through an attunement, we can start to isolate thoughts and attitudes, looking at them with fresh eyes. Through this we may choose to rethink an idea or attitude thus creating a new experience. The mental body seeks to create what it believes to be true and thus the healing implications for it are immense. The third attunement clarifies, aligns and clears this layer supporting a re-patterning; it brings the mental body into a more harmonious relationship with the cosmos.

Third Chakra ~ Solar plexus

The solar plexus chakra is the centre of our personal fire, and governs digestion and assimilation of events. Fire can nourish, warm, eliminate or burn. What we process through our chakra system through prana, food and life's experiences can nourish, sustain and illuminate our minds and hearts.

On a physical level this centre rules the stomach region, metabolic rate, gallbladder, liver and the nervous system.

People who find it challenging to express their deeper emotions can often suffer from increased symptoms of stomach ulcers, problems with digestion and nerves. This can be the way their body is indicating that there is a problem. We digest our emotions through this area of our body and solar plexus. If we cannot for some reason digest or process emotions we can create a charge in particular in the abdomen and internal organs. Left unprocessed these charges can impact upon our well- being and long term health.

On an emotional level this chakra deals with issues of personal power. People who have too much fire passing though this centre can experience the need to dominate others, can become easily irritable or quickly angry.

People who have low fire energy passing through this chakra can experience low self-worth, insecurity and may find it difficult to make decisions.

The third attunement plays a supportive role in balancing our fire energy. It is attuned to either bring more fire into the solar plexus or draw out any overactive fire.

The third attunement also encourages us to realize and know that the same power that creates and shapes the universe flows through us. We are not the source of power but the conduit and from this perspective we are constantly replenished in the flow of creation.

The third attunement carries another quality for this chakra. The attunement can align our consciousness to one of abundance and plenty. It does this through the combined energies of Citrine and Amber which are both warming, replenishing and nurturing. With the energies of Citrine and Amber we experience the activity of Citrine and the restfulness of Amber. This can teach us much about abundance, that it is best appreciated through the balancing energies of action and rest. When these two forces combine within us we can take the action needed to create abundance yet also know when to rest and appreciate what we have created.

The Oversouls for the Third Attunement

There are two Oversouls aligned to this attunement. They are yin and yang, Amber being the more inward calming yin, Citrine the more outward extrovert yang. To me it makes perfect sense that these two qualities are in a continual flux within us and therefore influence this attunement.

Amber has a warming energy that comforts and encourages us to take care of our power. We are conduits of immense spiritual energies that seek expression via our bodies. If we push ourselves too hard and don't allow time for rest and relaxation, or time to allow energies to be assimilated by our body, it is the solar plexus chakra that can become burnt out. This can lead to a breakdown in the delicate etheric web surrounding the stomach area of the body. This in turn affects the pranic energy being processed by organs around the stomach region, leading to a drop in overall energy levels and tiredness. Amber encourages us to listen to our body's signals and needs – to rest when need be and trust more in the timing of of life.

Citrine is a master teacher on the qualities of abundance and wealth. Whatever we need for the completion of our mission in life is potentially available to us, we just need to learn how to accept it and learn in what form it may come. Abundance is a state of being, a feeling and it is free to all. Citrine reminds us that the world is a generous, joyous and bountiful place and that we can participate in this abundance if we choose to. Our energy field oscillates at a frequency that reflects our beliefs. This crystal teaches us that what we believe will come into our reality. Citrine asks us to examine what we believe about life, to learn to raise the standard of our expectations with an open heart and mind.

The Crystals for the Third Attunement

All of these crystals fit within the framework of the third attunement. You could choose all from the list and place them in your circle. Alternatively choose one crystal that appeals to you, build a mandala and place the crystal in the centre. Or choose a few from the list that appeal, placing them throughout the circle. There are no rules so be creative and trust yourself.

Lemurian Golden Healer has a distinctive golden hue that is created through a wash of iron hydrate on or near the surface. It is a master crystal, radiating the golden ray of wisdom, balance and assimilation into our auric field.

Lemurian Golden Healer helps us navigate through the many personal changes taking place, as well as the Earth's shifting direction. This crystal reminds us to trust in our inherent power, to believe in the future and to embrace change.

Many of us are here at the critical stage in human evolution with much of our Lemurian DNA intact. With the assistance of this crystal, the part of our DNA that remembers Lemuria is activated. Ancient layers of our DNA start to awaken, restoring codes that will assist our journey. These memories carry the seeds that will assist us in this lifetime. The third attunement encourages us to embrace our wisdom and power by aligning us to ancient forces lain dormant within.

We are reminded of our powerful light that radiates throughout our being, and that we have no need to fear others response to this light. The time is perfect for us to shine, being true to our divine powers, sharing them with a world that is open and ready to accept our vastness.

Citrine is truly placed to support our journey to wholeness. Abundance in all its forms is our birthright. Our solar plexus, being the seat of our power is perfectly capable of remembering how to create a life of genuine wealth and well-being. Citrine reminds us of the joyous light that oversees and sustains us. Through the third attunement we are encouraged to remember, to allow, and surrender to the goodness that seeks our happiness.

We can, if we choose to, feel safe in the knowledge that universal forces desire to bless and sustain our well-being.

Gold Tektite has an extremely important position in the third attunement. Deep within the matrix of the Earth Star chakra are stored ancient seeds. These seeds contain our Lemurian stories of power. These seeds await the light of a new age to awaken them from their slumber. The third attunement is part of this awakening. When these seeds ripen they spill out their stories in the form of codes. These codes then surge into two lines of light that rise up from the Earth Star on their way towards the solar plexus chakra.

These lines weave their way around the base and sacral chakras, clearing the pathways of any distorted power issues that may still remain from previous lives. Once at the solar plexus the lines start to restore the energy of the solar plexus, offering a new template of compassion and power. Past life memories of misuse or loss of power that may have been stored in the solar plexus can be replaced by a new feeling of warmth, self worth, vitality, optimism and the sheer joy of living.

Amblygonite is a perfect balancer for the solar plexus centre. This chakra is the seat of our power. It can become disturbed by stress and anxiety which if left unaddressed can lead to a disturbance in our fire energy. We need our fire energy to burn away dross and that which is no longer necessary for our well-being. When we apply Amblygonite within the third attunement we begin to experience feelings of contentment and deep peace. All we approach is imbued with calm and ease.

Faden quartz is a unique find in the quartz family. It appears as a tabular crystal formation with a thread of white running through its centre. Faden quartz supports us through its ability to connect and thread energies together. If we apply Faden quartz within the third attunement, we can experience a powerful Soul connection.

Each of us is born with a silver umbilical cord that connects us to our Soul. This silver cord remains intact throughout our lifetime, serving as a source of subtle communication between our Soul and subconscious mind. Its roots and point of connection is at the solar plexus chakra. With some people this silver cord can become damaged through traumatic events in their present or past lives. If this is the case then Faden quartz steps up to assist us in the sacred reconnection of our cord. Through the third attunement we are guided to the point or memory where the disconnection occurred and loving assists in restoring our connection.

Amber is a fossilized tree resin that when applied to healing reminds us to relax. With all the transformation and initiations in this lifetime we can lose sight of the importance of integration and relaxation. The process of integration can challenge us as it asks us to let go, to be and allow for times of doing nothing. This process is deceptive though as what looks like nothing on the surface is in actuality an important part of our journey. The path to wholeness is a balance of action and resting. What is taking place under the surface of our being is in reality very active and alive. This process needs us to rest and allow it to take its time. Amber seeks to assist this part of our journey.

Stellar Beam calcite is a form of golden, amber or yellow calcite with long sharp terminations at either end. When we apply Stellar Beam Calcite within the framework of the third attunement, we can begin to open our imagination to the infinite possibilities contained within our being, and the cosmos. We can blend and merge our consciousness within the vast network of the Divine mind, giving us access to vast fields of information.

This beautiful crystal has a powerful restorative effect within the fine membrane of our mental body through its ability to help us to face outdated attitudes that no longer reflect our higher consciousness. Stellar Beam Calcite helps us dispel thought forms that we may have inherited or picked up from others. These thought forms attach themselves to the mental body's fine membrane. This can have the effect of sending signals to the mental body that could be unhealthy.

When we merge our consciousness with this crystal we can begin to release, through the inherent wisdom of our being, thought forms that do not reflect our vastness. We can then begin to imagine a new updated script that reflects more of our vastness.

The Fourth Attunement

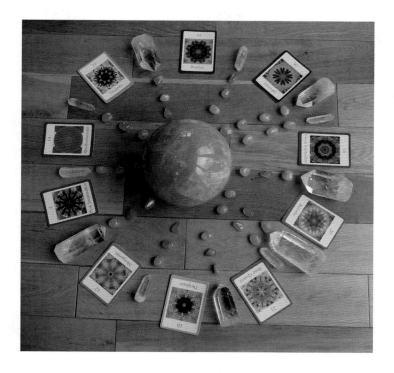

Mandala for the Fourth Attunement: as long as all the Crystal Oversoul cards mentioned are used, feel free to add any or all of the crystals mentioned. In the above picture I have added a Rose quartz as well as many quartz points. If a crystal is added to your mandala, make sure you read what that particular crystal will bring into your attunement.

Crystals: Rose Quartz, Cobalto Calcite, Dioptase, Emerald, Green Heulandite, Jade, Kunzite, Hiddenite, Lithium in quartz, Malachite, Morganite, Rhodochrosite, Seriphos, Tugtupite, Green Tourmaline, Pink Tourmaline, Peridot.

Crystal Oversoul cards: Peridot, Emerald, Green Tourmaline, Kunzite, Rose quartz, Dioptase, Morganite, Pink Tourmaline, Rhodochrosite, Vivianite.

Overview

Chakra Subject: Connection, compassion, inner joy.

Body position: Centre of chest.

Organs & glands: Lungs, heart, breath, thymus, skin, upper chest, ribs and shoulders.

Tree of life position: Upper arc of Tiphareth.

Colours: Green or pink

Musical Note: F

Seed syllable: Yam

Archangel: Michael

Element: Air

The fourth attunement has its primary focus on the astral body and heart chakra. The Crystal Oversoul temples of Peridot, Emerald, Green Tourmaline, Kunzite, Rose quartz, Dioptase, Morganite, Pink Tourmaline, Rhodochrosite and Vivianite combine forces to activate, attune and strengthen the astral body as well as the heart chakra. If we also add any of the crystals; Rose Quartz, Cobalto Calcite, Dioptase, Emerald, Green Heulandite, Jade, Kunzite, Hiddenite, Lithium in quartz, Malachite, Morganite, Rhodochrosite, Seriphos, Tugtupite, Green Tourmaline, Pink Tourmaline and Peridot we have an attunement that is made up of a vast range of attunements within attunements.

Layout for the Fourth Attunement

If you resonate with this attunement read the following writing first. Familiarize yourself with as much of the information as possible. You can do this process as many times as you like. Each time will be different because it affects another moment of your journey.

Decide if you are to lie sit or stand within the mandala.

Lay the named crystal Oversoul cards in a mandala matching the position of your body.

Choose any of the mentioned crystals or all of them. All the ones you choose will be drawn into the energetic mixture. Another option is to decide different quantities of the same stone, for example, two Kunzite. Be creative and trust your intuition. Lay these crystals within the Oversoul mandala.

Once your mandala is laid out, lay or stand inside the mandala. The crystal Oversoul cards provide a gateway for the energy necessary to protect, open and offer the created space for the attunement. Relax, resting with the support of the crystal consciousness and its innate ability to transport you to the level and frequency that is correct for you. There is nothing you need to direct. The more you relax and allow, the deeper the process can become.

It is difficult to say for how long the process lasts as this work has a time all of its own. An obvious drop in energy can be felt when the process is complete.

Fourth Auric layer

Astral — *Element:* Air

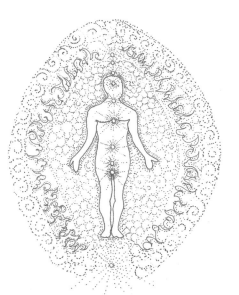

As we move, extend our awareness even further outwards from the mental body, we move into the realm of the astral body. This body extends itself outwards by a few feet.

The astral body serves as a bridge between the lower bodies; physical, etheric, emotional and mental. It is through this body that we astral travel.

We astral travel during many experiences such as imagining, sleeping, dreaming and fantasising.

When we undertake inner work such as therapy and counselling we use our astral body to retrace steps in our memory. The astral body is also active during journey work such as shamanism, guided journeys, pathworking and trance meditation.

This body also has what is known as a silver cord, connecting us, via the astral body, to the upper bodies of soul and spirit.

The astral body is a bridge between the higher octaves of our being, our etheric double upwards. It acts as a conductor of the incoming imprints of the higher bodies and translates these impulses into the lower bodies of mental and emotional. These bodies then adapt the incoming information by translating it according to balance, where needed.

The attunements in this book are the obvious vehicle for the astral body. Whenever we slip out of everyday consciousness it is the astral body that travels and gathers information. The fourth attunement assists us by aligning our astral body to a higher consciousness awareness. When this sheath of our being is returned from the attunement it has been altered to take on the higher light of new DNA patterns. When we return into our physical body awareness these patterns are re-absorbed into our auric system and thus change begins.

The astral body is also used by the higher bodies to communicate to lower bodies. If, say, the soul body wishes to impart information it will call out the astral body and impregnate it with information. This can sometimes lead to odd feelings when this happens during our waking state, as if we are not all there, and in effect we are not. At times like this it can be best to rest and wait until the astral body returns. I often have this experience when writing. If I do not know something and know that my being does, I will send out my astral body to ask my higher bodies the question.

More often than not the answer arrives in minutes. If I get really stuck on a question I do this before going to sleep. I always wake up with the answer.

I also use this process with the crystal Oversouls themselves. If I want to ask them something it is my astral body which seeks out their guidance. This process is simple now but when I first encountered the Oversouls my astral body was often overwhelmed by their energy.

When I guide a group to meet an Oversoul during a meditation it takes my astral body quite some time to adjust on my return. Although I travel in my own astral body during these meditations I also carry within this sheath the astral bodies of those in my keeping. Until the others are back in their physical awareness they are under my protection.

The astral body is very sensitive to images and impressions. If for example we observe violence and negative images in a film it is the astral body that feels and believes the images to be true. Obviously we need to be careful what we watch and what we believe.

Another important function of the astral body is its involvement with the turn in evolution that we are currently experiencing. During our sleeping state our astral bodies are working, depending on our abilities and functions, with many others assisting the process of awakening. When this works well we do not remember when we wake – when there is a lot of activity on the astral we wake up with a vague sensation that we have been involved in conflicts and sometimes real horrors.

Humanity plays out many of its dramas in the world on the physical plane. However it also plays out the same dramas on a much wider level on the astral plane and it is in the struggle of forces, both within humanity and also in the cosmos that do not want humanity to change, that many beings get caught up in. These forces resist humanity raising itself to a new vibration and interfere. Many beings work alongside unseen beings of light to bring about a new age. They experience and are really involved in this conflict between the forces of change and the forces of suppression on the astral.

This fourth attunement can help to clarify our conscious knowledge of the astral body. When we work with this body with its intended functions we open ourselves to infinite possibilities.

Fourth Chakra ~ Heart

The heart chakra relates to our thymus in the centre of our chest. The thymus, being an element of the immune system and endocrine system, plays an important role in the protection and maintenance of our well-being. If we become stressed this is the centre that can become most affected.

This chakra governs many of our emotions ranging from love and compassion to jealousy and hatred. On the ladder of the chakras we are at the middle point where we start to travel above our human self up into a sense of connection to a bigger picture.

There are 17 crystals and 10 Oversouls that serve as ambassadors of the heart chakra.

I was intrigued when writing this part of the book about the intense focus of the Oversouls on this attunement. They combine forces for many of the attunements, but much moreso for this one. When I asked the Oversouls about the Heart they showed me a picture of Peridot, Emerald, Green Tourmaline, Kunzite, Rose quartz, Dioptase, Morganite, Pink Tourmaline, Rhodochrosite and Vivianite Oversouls, all merging into a mandala of exquisite geometry.

I found it difficult to comprehend how they could do this as well as joining forces with the crystals Rose Quartz, Cobalto Calcite, Dioptase, Emerald, Green Heulandite, Jade, Kunzite, Hiddenite, Lithium in quartz, Malachite, Morganite, Rhodochrosite, Seriphos, Tugtupite, Green Tourmaline, Pink Tourmaline and Peridot. To me this combination implies prior knowledge on their part in the attunement and initiation of the heart.

It shows how much potential the heart carries in our journey to wholeness, not only in this life but in many others. The following discourse is from the Oversouls:

"Within the chambers of the heart chakra rests a sacred flame. This flame is contained within an inner temple upon an altar. This sacred flame is maintained throughout incarnated life through inner work. The flame serves as a reflection of inner life. It cannot go out, but it can appear to dwindle. The fourth attunement is designed to support all that can be learnt about this flame. Through its light much can be learnt about oneself."

I have taken groups on guided meditations to meet this flame. On many of these journeys people have experienced that their flame is in a dusty temple that has not been visited for aeons. However their symbolic scenario does not indicate that we cannot change things. Through our heart presence and awareness the temple can be aired and become alive. We can tend to the flame by giving it permission to illuminate again.

For this attunement read through the crystal list. Apply the one or ones that are most appropriate to your subject putting those within the grid. If you are drawn to place all within the grid then do so.

The Oversouls for the Fourth Attunement

There are ten Oversouls aligned with this attunement. It fits, I feel, that there are ten as the heart chakra is a pivotal place within our system. When I was first researching this book I started to meditate with each of the 44 Oversouls, to ask which ones were aligned with which attunement. When I was meditating on the fourth attunement I was overwhelmed by the amount of Oversouls that came forwards, expressing their positions in this mandala.

Peridot signifies the end of a long cycle and the beginning of another. The cycle about to end will draw away that which no longer can serve our highest good, clearing the path for more potential to manifest. At times like this Peridot comes into its own and helps to stay strong and generous, enabling us to stay focused on the positive energies available to us.

Peridot comes as the gift after the storm, the blessing of peace, abundance and hope.

The heart chakra can be cleansed with this crystal. This leads the way to a deeper and more refined access to one's personal energies. Peridot is a particular healing companion for those who have a tendency to turn their power against themselves when in distress or confusion.

The heart chakra is attuned to the deep green ray offered by **Emerald**. Blockages that we allow to stand in the way of achieving our dreams are reflected back to us.

The Emerald Oversoul takes us to the roots of any residual feelings connected to how we value ourselves. Emerald asks us to look within and to ask penetrating questions as to the nature of our reality. Rather than prematurely blaming or judging another for our experience, Emerald asks us to first seek healing around our own attitude.

All real healing starts with the willingness to change, and this crystal supports us in moving forward into the unknown regions of the heart, giving us courage, strength and ultimately true wealth. Within this inner movement we can discover how precious we are.

Green Tourmaline is a wonderful tonic for the heart. The energies of this crystal can rebuild an exhausted or closed heart chakra. The subtle green ray emanating from this stone asks us to remain fresh and renewed in the moment, to let go of any past misunderstandings and be present to what is here and now.

Green Tourmaline helps us remember our soul mission by taking us to the heart of the dream that we nurture within. Through this experience an awakening occurs and the song that resides in our soul's heart starts to sing. If we learn to listen and follow our soul's song we will be guided ever deeper.

Kunzite is an important healing companion as it encourages us to relax and take each step at a time, to come into the moment and accept life for what it is, not what we think it should be.

Sometimes in life we need action and determination to make things happen and sometimes we need to let go and let the universe handle the details. Kunzite comes into its own under these circumstances. Its soft and powerful light reminds us on a deep level to trust in our inner process, that all is well and will unfold for our deepest good.

Kunzite activates in us a deep appreciation of life, reminding us that the universe is a benevolent and loving force that seeks the best for us, if we allow it.

Rose Quartz is a gentle but firm guide through the journey of uncovering the past. It supports the heart chakra to open like a flower – revealing petal after petal. There is nothing rushed about this journey – step by step. Rose quartz is an excellent tonic for people who are judged by others or by themselves as over sensitive. The vibrations of Rose quartz can help dissolve walls of self protection and fear. Through this process, sensitivity and vulnerability are exposed. It helps to realize these powerful feelings, to protect oneself and still be open to the world and others.

Rose quartz is a very feminine crystal; it encourages us to

live our sensitivity with openness and honour. Our energy field then radiates these qualities without any compromise.

Dioptase is a powerful healer for the heart, thymus, nerves, lower lungs and chest region. The heart chakra processes and gathers energy in this area. If there is a disturbance or upset in the balance of energy this chakra cannot function properly and thus our overall health can suffer. The disturbances can be holding on to grievances, guilt, envy and dwelling on upsets or not airing our feelings. By working with Dioptase we can learn to express any feelings that we do not wish to hold onto and do not serve our health.

Dioptase has a fresh optimistic healing vibration that will have a positive influence on our whole sense of well-being. It is a stone of cleansing and new beginnings.

Morganite is a master healer encouraging us to heal feelings of separation. As a healing companion this crystal asks us to merge with what we are resisting. Morganite's vibration encourages us to take our needs and ourselves seriously, to know that we are creating our well-being through our actions. If reality is not what we want, we need to seek out what it is we do need to change, to achieve an improvement.

Morganite supports introspection and examination of what our feelings want to communicate. We have great potential and wisdom in our emotions and this power can go for us or against us. Morganite benefits those who find they can be easily overwhelmed by feelings, be it their own or another's.

Pink Tourmaline encourages us to let go, to relax. To forgive when we can and make space for love. With pink tourmaline the heart chakra can be unburdened of residue, letting in fresh energy and optimism.

Grace, respect and love are the key words for pink tourmaline. This crystal encourages openness and trust in life. It asks us to remain true to our inner guidance and to seek validation from our knowing, rather than another. Pink tourmaline initiates strength and communication with the heart.

Patterns around love, sharing and responsibility for our feelings are addressed through this crystal. This crystal's soft healing pink tones the physical body, relaxes and releases any tension.

Rhodochrosite is a sacred healer for the heart chakra, signalling that it is time to arise from the past. Patterns that have inhibited confidence and joy for life are revealed and – if you are ready – released.

It asks us to remember that we are the physical manifestation and expression of our soul's light here on earth. It encourages us to learn to play and enjoy life, to celebrate the goodness and sweetness of all the earth has to offer. The divine spark flows through our veins and if we have forgotten this, Rhodochrosite serves to remind us. During meditation or healing you can call upon the energies of this wise crystal, helping you awaken to love's presence.

Vivianite serves to remind us of the strength and generosity of our hearts. Its energies help us shift feelings of resentment and fear from the heart and solar plexus chakras. These feelings, if left unaddressed, can weigh down our life force. Through this energy release we can find the compassion of our being and face anything.

Vivianite is a powerful healing ally that when meditated with or carried reminds us of our inner strength and our innate ability to let go of any feelings that are inhibiting the deepest expression of our life force.

Vivianite's message is that life is too short to hold onto grudges or to keep putting things off: 'Face that which needs to be done and start the journey to your personal fulfillment'.

The Crystals for the Fourth Attunement

All of these crystals fit within the framework of the fourth attunement. You could choose all from the list and place them in your circle. Alternatively choose one crystal that appeals to you, build a mandala and place the crystal in the centre. Or choose a few from the list that appeal, placing them throughout the circle. There are no rules so be creative and trust yourself.

Rose quartz when applied during the fourth attunement stimulates a gentle opening and strengthening of the heart. During the ceremony this simple yet elegant crystal gently supports a repairing of the heart chakra. If we are carrying residues of past hurts and resentments it is the heart chakra where these feelings reside. They can if left unaddressed corrode our life force taking the joy of the moment away from our experience of life. When we apply Rose quartz in this attunement we are supported in a new way of feeling about ourselves and the past. We are reminded that although we cannot change the past we can change our attitude to it.

A further aspect to the application of Rose quartz during this attunement is that we are reminded of the infinite depth of love we carry within ourselves. We can remember that we are the source of the love which we seek. We need no other to satisfy our desire for love and acceptance as we can fulfil these feelings for ourself. Rose quartz is a true master in the mineral kingdom, simple yet deep and profound. When we allow ourselves to be taken under its wings we can learn much about ourselves and our attitude to the past.

Cobalto Calcite (also known as **Pink Dolomite**) is a beautiful crystal that when we encounter its presence encourages us to let go of fear, relax, trust and breathe into our deepest being. The deep warm pink colour that this crystal exhibits seems to relax the eye of the beholder. When we apply this crystal within the context of the fourth attunement we become more open and responsive to healing, in particular within the region of the astral body.

Our astral body is the conductor, the translator of information being imparted from the higher levels of our aura. If our astral body becomes restricted through fear this important layer of our being is unable to filter any incoming messages. These messages could assist us in our healing and if we are closed off to them we are closing off an important channel of communication between our conscious awareness and our higher self.

Dioptase: during the fourth attunement we are assisted, through welcoming this crystal into our awareness, into a powerful process whereby we are brought into the moment, unburdened by past life misunderstandings. Our astral body can become burdened and occupied by past life and karmic patterns. If this is the case we may find that whatever inner healing work we do it does not become reality for us. If this is the case it can be that we need to look to our astral body for healing. During this attunement, with Dioptase as our guide, we are able to release our attachment to the past and set ourselves free. This being the case the astral body can then take on board new patterns that we choose to believe as it is unburdened by the past. What our astral body believes becomes our reality.

Emerald is an important ally in our journey to wholeness. If we have a tendency to make ourselves small by hiding our light, we are doing a dis-service to our vast potential. The deep green rays of this crystal penetrate our resistance to our vastness, illuminating the voices within us that believe we are unworthy of such beauty. Through this attunement we meet these voices through imagery and imagination. We start to understand where the roots of our unworthiness first took hold. Through this we can start to move into a deep compassion for ourselves that expands and unfolds our heart.

Green Heulandite exhibits a soft earthy green colour. In the fourth attunement we are guided by this crystal to connect and feel the heartbeat of the Earth. This sacred attunement gently asks us to see life and humanity through the eyes of the Earth. From this perspective we begin to comprehend the movement of time and human history. We are invited to feel for our fellow human travellers as well as compassion for our own journey.

When we invite **Jade** into the attunement process with us we are asking to become more conscious of our sacred dream. Each of us carries an ancient dream that needs the right conditions to emerge. For many the time of emergence is now. By working with Jade within this framework we first hear our dream as a whisper. We are encouraged to take time to nurture our dream, to get to know it, to understand what will be required.

Through this we will know what action to take and what we may need to let go of to give it space. This attunement encourages us to keep quiet, at this stage, to let our dream gradually unfold through nurturing these early embryonic stages.

When we welcome **Kunzite** into the fourth attunement we are asking to learn all we can about trust. Most of all, regaining trust in ourselves via our intuition. The soft lilac pink colour rays that Kunzite exhibits is deeply nurturing and balancing upon the heart and third eye chakras. Through the balancing of these powerful energy centres we enter a powerful stage in our development – a deep knowing of what is right for us. This can serve us well in our unfolding as we start to trust our intuition as our guide and navigation through uncertain times.

Hiddenite is a variety of spodumene and is also known as **Green Kunzite** and **Lithia Emerald**. Hiddenite exhibits a soft green colour that encourages us to open our heart and trust others. This crystal plays an important place in our healing journey as it supports reconciliation and connection. Our heart chakra is the centre whereby we connect and inter-act.

If we have been hurt by others we may have closed off this chakra to protect ourselves. Although understandable, if we block off any chakra we will be restricting our life force.

During this attunement we are reminded that we need others to support our development, that we are here together to expand and unfold our light.

Another aspect that can be addressed during this attunement with Hiddenite is the need to control. If we seek to control others, and life, we will become distressed. During this attunement we are supported in letting go of the reigns of control bit by bit.

Lithium in quartz is as the name suggests natural lithium that appears as a lilac coloured phantom in quartz. The qualities of lithium are further amplified through their being in quartz. This mineral has a balancing, nurturing and supportive presence that can play a part in the treatment of depression, fear and anxiety. Depression, fear and anxiety can all restrict our life force rendering some incapable of functioning. When we create the mandala for the fourth attunement we create a space whereby Lithium in quartz offers its services in clearing from within the heart and third eye any accumulated energy that is impeding our life-force.

Malachite appears twice in the attunements. Firstly in the first attunement and again, here in the fourth. Much of what has been offered in this book concerns the dreams that we carry within our being. In this attunement Malachite is the heart and dream protector - the space giver. Once we have got to know our dream, explored and realized it we will at some point wish to give it space in the world. Our dream will need to be born. This is Malachite's strength.

When we work with it in this attunement process we are given the protection that our dream will need, especially at the early stages. If we seek to become visible, unfolding our dream into the world we will need to inhabit some degree of space.

Malachite supports this process by encouraging us to expand, to move forwards and create with confidence in our abilities.

Morganite (also known as **Pink Beryl** or **Pink Emerald**) exhibits an exquisite soft pink colour that restores harmony and balance to our being. The tender pink rays of this crystal direct themselves into our heart chakra, astral and emotional bodies by way of direct healing transference. What is being received by us balances a particular area of our life - our ability to give and receive. If we put others first and exhaust our own reserves, this can be balanced. If we are self-absorbed, unable to read other peoples' needs, this too is balanced.

Rhodochrosite is a master of the heart being able to teach us much about living fully present on Earth with a positive image of ourself. When we combine this powerful crystal within this attunement we are calling upon great healing potential. We can, if we are willing during this process, release any feelings of lack of self-worth and damaging images we have taken on board. Within this attunement we are deeply supported in letting go of negative images we have accepted and believed to be true. We are offered a more honest, loving, accepting impression that reflects who we really are.

Seriphos green quartz (also known as **Prasem**) is found in one location; a small Greek Island called Seriphos. Seriphos green quartz is an infusion of Hedenbergite minerals which give this crystal a green leaf like colouring. When we welcome Seriphos into our attunement we are ready to embrace an abundant, joy filled life. This crystal assists us in releasing out dated beliefs that life is or should be a struggle and burden. We are encouraged to challenge what we believe, to be ready to connect, via our heart, with the joy of life.

Tugtupite assists in a very important process of our journey. Some carry ancient sorrow within the ancient chambers of the heart. These sorrows can have many roots, one of them being the pain of humanity. If we have had past lives where we have seen much suffering and hardship we may be carrying these feelings deep within our heart. Tugtupite is unique in its ability to guide us towards these sorrows if these are inhibiting our life force in this life time. Through this attunement we are taken to the core of our heart and asked if we still wish to hold onto these feelings or let them go. Tugtupite is a powerful crystalline being that radiates an intense penetrating clarity. Combined within the protective space of an attunement this crystal is perfectly suited to assist us on our journey to wholeness.

Green Tourmaline is a beautiful tonic for Soul and heart. When we work with this crystal during the fourth attunement we begin to magnify our experience on Earth. Through this process Green Tourmaline helps us remember our Soul mission. Our Soul has a plan that requires the right environment and set of events for it to be realized. We all carry within our heart the template of this plan that only we, along with our Soul's support, can nurture it into manifestation. During this attunement we are supported in not only remembering but also giving birth to our Soul's mission.

Pink Tourmaline is a powerful crystalline companion that puts us in touch with our bliss. The colours can range from soft rose to deep fuchsia pink, and can be beautiful upon the eye and heart. When we apply this crystal within the fourth attunement we are inviting highly refined energies to work alongside us, helping us to find our bliss, to free our heart. During the attunement we are invited to release restrictive energies that may be inhibiting the flow of our life force. We are reminded that in the free movement of the heart we are freer than we sometimes allow.

Peridot: when we ask this beautiful crystal to participate in our mandala we are asking for a release of anything that no longer serves our highest good. Peridot is a combination of green and gold rays, signifying harmony between the solar plexus and heart chakras. When these two chakras are in alignment our power and knowing are perfectly balanced enabling us to move forward in absolute clarity. The fourth attunement supports our light in unfolding free from any hindrance of the past. We are supported by Peridot in letting go and stepping confidently into the new.

The Fifth Attunement

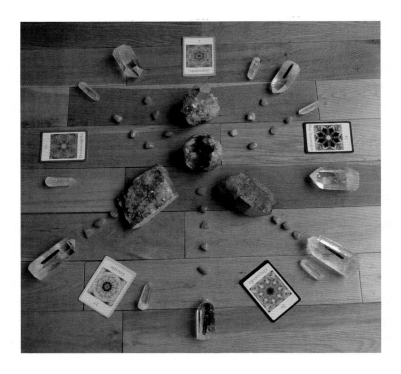

Mandala for the Fifth Attunement: as long as all the Crystal Oversoul cards mentioned are used feel free to add any or all of the crystals mentioned. In the above picture I have added a Ajoite, Celestite, Kyanite and Aquamarine as well as many quartz points. If a crystal is added to your mandala, make sure you read what that particular crystal will bring into your attunement.

Crystals: Blue Tourmaline quartz, Ajoite, Hemimorphite, Chrysocolla, Celestite, Amazonite, Aquamarine, Blue Apatite, Larimar, Kyanite.

Crystal Oversoul cards: Aquamarine, Blue Tourmaline, Chrysocolla, Celestite, Hemimorphite.

Overview

Chakra Subject: Expression & Confidence.

Chakra Body Position: Throat.

Organ & glands: Thyroid, ears, nose, throat, lungs, neck and respiratory system.

Tree of life position: Lower arc of Daath.

Colour: Blue

Musical Note: G

Seed syllable: Ham

Archangel: Michael

Element: Ether

The fifth attunement has its primary focus on the etheric template and throat chakra. The Crystal Oversoul temples of Aquamarine, Blue Tourmaline, Chrysocolla, Celestite and Hemimorphite combine forces to activate, attune and strengthen the etheric template as well as the throat chakra.

If we also add any of the crystals; Blue Tourmaline, Turquoise, Blue phantom quartz, Ajoite, Hemimorphite, Chrysocolla, Celestite, Amazonite, Aquamarine, Blue Apatite, Larimar, Kyanite, we have an attunement that opens up our journey even further.

Layout for the Fifth Attunement

If you resonate with this attunement read the following writing first. Familiarize yourself with as much of the information as possible. You can do this process as many times as you like. Each time will be different because it affects another moment of your journey.

Decide if you are to lie within the mandala, sit or stand.

Lay the named crystal Oversoul cards in a mandala matching the position of your body.

Choose any of the mentioned crystals or all of them. All the ones you choose will be drawn into the energetic mixture. Another option is to decide different quantities of the same stone, for example, six Aquamarine. Be creative and trust your intuition. Lay these crystals within the Oversoul mandala.

Once your mandala is laid out lay or stand inside the mandala. The crystal Oversoul cards provide a gateway for the energy necessary to protect, open and offer the created space for the attunement. Relax, resting with the support of the crystal consciousness and its innate ability to transport you to the level and frequency that is correct for you. There is nothing you need to direct. The more you relax and allow, the deeper the process can become.

It is difficult to say for how long the process lasts as this work has a time all of its own. An obvious drop in energy can be felt when the process is complete.

Fifth Auric layer

Etheric Template – *Element:* Ether

From this level onwards we are nurtured and sustained by quite different forces. The etheric template carries the patterning that will serve our existence in incarnated life. This template will store all of the karmic patterns that we need to gain our experiences on earth, in our body. The template looks like a holo-

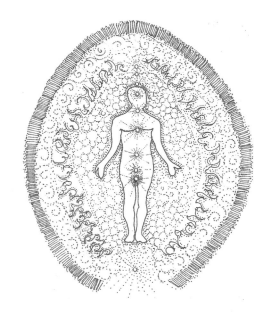

gram of vibrant blue webbed light that extends around all of the lower four bodies. This body of light looks rather like an ethereal scaffolding or an architect's drawing, which gives a clue as to its functions.

What we have decided upon before incarnating will be stored within this body. All the potential people we shall meet, all the lessons that could be learned and all the learning that could take place is carried in this body.

It changes from life to life depending on what we do with the information at hand. When I look at this layer I see the miracle of exquisite design start to unfold. There is an infinite amount of intelligence contained within this body.

All we are to be, to become and develop into is there to see as a potential. This is an important aspect to explore: All is *potential* that seeks to be explored. We can explore this consciously through inner and practical work, or leave the potential unconscious. However unconscious, this energy will seek ways to get our attention. That could be through illness, depression, crisis or other ways of making us turn towards what it is that is seeking our attention. Perhaps this energy will remain unexplored in this body until the next life.

We explore this layer mainly through inner work. By that I refer to meditation, past life regression, counselling or other forms of self-development. The fifth attunement encourages us to know that we are the same consciousness that creates the template of our experiences, therefore we can explore the potential for other realities other than the one presenting itself to us.

The fifth attunement also allows us to traverse the physical, etheric, emotional, mental and astral bodies, propelling our consciousness into the etheric template's landscape. This is the sheath of the aura where we immerse our light in the plane of bliss. Encountering bliss sounds very nice and has enormous healing potential because once we have experienced and remembered bliss a shift in consciousness needs to take place that changes us forever.

Our returning consciousness travels back through all of our other sheaths; astral, mental, emotional, etheric and physical with the experience of bliss intact. Our cells become drenched in the returning blissful light, forever altered. Through the fifth attunement we also become conscious that we are far larger than we had previously imagined.

Fifth Chakra ~ Throat

The throat chakra is positioned over the throat and neck region. It governs speech, confidence, fears, hearing, intuition and creativity.

A balanced throat chakra is enhanced by keeping the lines of communication open between others and ourselves. It is important to maintain this chakra's health and well-being by expressing our feelings. It is just as important to talk about things when they are going well as it is to talk about our hurts, anxieties and vulnerability.

We are unique spiritual beings that desire to express this quality in the world. With the support of all other levels of our being we desire to have our uniqueness honoured.

Historically, humanity does not tend to support outsiders or uniqueness. The key to dealing with this, I find, is not to try and fit in but to stay true to our nature and let humanity fit into us. The fifth attunement offers us a new reality or template whereby we stand tall in our uniqueness. With this attitude we are able to express our inner vision within the world.

If we have had challenging past lives where we were persecuted for expressing our beliefs or we were different, this can be the chakra most affected in the form of restrictive energy trapped within the chakra, mirrored also on the etheric template.

The fifth attunement helps us unwind any restrictions within the core of the chakra that still holds on to memories of persecution. Through letting these feelings go we are able to move forward, letting the universe support our feelings of acceptance and openness.

It is the throat chakra which carries memories of lack, restriction and suffering. If we experience anything other than a deeply supportive universal system that supplies all we need, then the fifth attunement will assist us. Through this attunement we start to experience a universe that seeks to give us everything we need to make our dreams come true, and we learn to know that we can accept this without guilt or fear of losing anything.

The throat chakra is also the point in our chakra system from where we cross over into the unknown regions of our being. From this point onwards we need the support of our intuition. The fifth attunement helps release any debris within the throat chakra that is still fearful or distrustful of our intuition. Through its alignment process we start to experience the serenity of our intuitive voice, letting us be guided from within.

The Oversouls for the Fifth Attunement

There are five Oversouls aligned with the fifth attunement. They are all shades of blue from dark to light, which seem perfectly placed to support this process. The numerology of number five means freedom, which aligns perfectly with this particular attunement.

Aquamarine: Collectively we are entering uncharted waters as a human race. The emotional body that has served as a blueprint of behaviour for the past two thousand years has completed itself. The next cycle of human history is already upon us and the emerging new layers of human consciousness are drawing the map. As we enter these multi-dimensional fields of possibilities, it is Aquamarine that is serving us in our adjustment.

Aquamarine is one of the most beneficial stones to call upon in times of need or upheaval. By working with this stone any fears or anxieties holding one back are brought to the surface.

Blue Tourmaline: This special crystal can take us deep into the silence within, as it is from silence that all ideas are eventually born. It is important for our general well-being to cultivate being-in-silence. Silence is a great healer and it has restorative effects on the mind and heart. When we return from silence we can look afresh at situations and solve problems that had previously held us back. Blue tourmaline balances the chakras around the throat, ears and eyes. All of these centres need to be in union for the state of silence to be entered. The inner planes, angels and inter-dimensional beings communicate through silence, so it stands to reason that if we desire communication we need to be able to listen.

Chrysocolla travels on the blue ray of communication, encouraging deep and heart-felt expression. It supports honesty in feelings and will support release of any tension in the throat chakra. Chrysocolla has a strong presence and asks us to express our vulnerability and sensitivity here on this earth. It puts us in touch with profound feminine qualities in ourselves. When this force is embraced we live connected to a powerful inner source of creativity and beauty and can express it in the world. Integrating our inner feminine and masculine power will play an increasingly important part in the development of humanity. Ultimately we are on the way to merging these inner male and female qualities where we are more complete in ourselves.

Celestite: As we enter a new stage of celestial and inter-dimensional contact we will be challenged to maintain our own spiritual integrity within the cosmos. This crystal encourages us to stand in the light of our knowing and to be able to discern what is right for us and what is not. This crystal has special connections to angelic forces. A subtle song inherent to its vibration can be heard when in its presence; this calls the angels and higher frequency beings to its side, which can offer complete protection and balance.

Celestite has a particular quality and resonance that can balance the throat chakra. It is this chakra which can need most healing if there has been a loss of faith or trust.

Hemimorphite: Our experience of life is reflected by the limits of our imagination. Hemimorphite stimulates a desire to explore the inner realms of our being and soar with our consciousness; to look at our situations from a higher perspective. We are taken on a journey to view life through the eyes of our soul and to keep things in perspective.

This crystal finds its way to people at a time in their life when a great awakening will take place. Hemimorphite is a guide, a physical manifestation of higher consciousness. It appears in a person's life to say 'wake up from your dream – the time you have been waiting for is here'. With this support we know that the time is right to move forward.

The Crystals for the Fifth Attunement

All of these crystals fit within the framework of the fifth attunement. You could choose all from the list and place them in your circle. Alternatively choose one crystal that appeals to you, build a mandala and place the crystal in the centre. Or choose a few from the list that appeal, placing them throughout the circle. There are no rules so be creative and trust yourself.

Blue Tourmaline: When used in conjunction with the fifth attunement this crystal supports the Blue Tourmaline Oversoul in its work to balance our aura at the level of the etheric template and throat chakra. The healing focus is to trust in the silence within. Silence is the gateway to our intuition. When we combine the Oversoul and crystal energy we are asking for a release of any restrictive patterns, be they karmic or from this life-time, that seek to inhibit our own connection to inner silence.

What we are seeking to remove from our path, when we partake in this attunement with Blue Tourmaline, is our own fear of authority or outside forces that we believe have power over us, thereby inhibiting our direct connection to our own intuition. Silence speaks a language that if we listen to it will guide us directly to our intuition. It is the sound and voice of our Soul.

Ajoite also appears in the eighth and ninth attunements being one of the most important evolutionary crystals for ascension. The best Ajoite comes from one location, the Messina mine in

South Africa, which is now closed due to the difficulties and dangers of the mine, which has collapsed making it impossible to enter safely.

Ajoite usually appears as an inclusion in quartz, an exquisite turquoise blue phantom. There can also be the presence of Hematite, Limonite and sometimes Papagoite. It is unlikely that any new sources of this rare crystal will come onto the market. I am intrigued by the rarity of certain stones, feeling that when a crystal becomes extinct or unavailable why would that be if these crystals want to assist in our healing journey. A possible explanation could be that this stone is so powerful that if it was freely available it could be overlooked or even abused.

Welcoming Ajoite into our mandala prepares us for an acceleration and quickening of our life force. When we work with Ajoite in this attunement we open ancient chambers in our throat chakra. These chambers have been inactive for thousands of years. As we enter a completely new cycle in human/galactic evolution we will need what is contained within these chambers. Inside are our sacred seals, our blueprints that we placed within ourselves in Lemuria for this lifetime, this time and space. Through this attunement we are issuing a call that we are ready to see and read what we sent to our future self that we would need to unfold our light.

Hemimorphite has a highly sought after vibration: it reminds us of the dream that we carry within our being. This dream will have a particular resonance with communication, the arts and creativity. The way I understand it, each of us carries a piece of the dream of humanity within the DNA of our being. Humanity will at some point need all of these pieces to come together as a scared jigsaw puzzle.

Hemimorphite triggers and activates the piece of the dream

that we carry sacred and protected within our being. If we are drawn to this crystal in particular it could indicate that we are ready to remember our part of the fragment of the dream. Simply add this crystal to your fifth attunement mandala and ask for support in remembering your dream. An interesting aspect of this is that when we awaken to our fragment of the dream the rest of the jigsaw notices and seeks to connect with us.

Chrysocolla is a true gift from the crystal devas. Its supportive energies envelop our energy field giving us beautiful feelings of safety and security. When we work with this crystal we can begin to explore how beautiful life on earth and our body can be. We are spiritual beings having a human experience – the human experience and living on earth can be one of profound beauty. This can be of a particular resonance with many souls around at this time as so many of us carry memories that challenge us to really enjoy our bodily incarnation with joy. When we welcome Chrysocolla into our attunement process we are asking to know the peace of our physical form. To learn to enjoy our body as a temple that houses our Light-body. We are welcoming beautiful, powerful, supportive energies of ease and grace into our life.

Celestite reminds us that every layer and fibre of our being is of divine creation. It elevates our consciousness to a higher plane of light and imagination where we become imbued with positive life affirming energy. If we have been feeling fearful, restricted or lacking in confidence the vibration of this crystal can help us become renewed and optimistic about life and all it offers. Meditation can open us up to many influences that exist on the inner and astral planes. Celestite plays a unique role in the fifth attunement as it strengthens our ability to discern what is right for our development. It offers us spiritual protection by wrapping us up its in cloak of Angelic light.

Amazonite supports our growth by reminding us just how strong we are and can be. Not, though, by being aggressive or forceful but through gentle strength that resides within. Amazonite helps us find the courage to make changes through speaking and clarifying our truth.

During the fifth attunement this special crystal plays an important role as it strengthens our ability to tell our story. By this I mean the story that only we can tell about the history and development of humanity. Each of us has been a witness to the stories the human race has experienced. Not all of these stories have been written in our history books or records. Over these next few years new and untold stories will emerge that will shine a new light on our past, most of all our origins. The fifth attunement along with Amazonite will enable us to communicate ancient stories, changing our perception of the past.

Aquamarine is derived from the latin words *aqua marina* meaning 'water of the sea'. It is a wonderful stone to be working with connecting us deeply to the water element. It is a major force in supporting us in discovering the wealth of feelings we have within our being. Through this we can, if we choose to, harness these feelings. Rather than be ashamed or frightened of our feelings we can learn to make something original out of them. When we apply Aquamarine in the fifth attunement we open not only our own psyche up for change but also humanity's.

Blue Apatite can have a cleansing and deeply healing effect on the etheric body, helping to purge outdated programmes and patterns. These can be ideas and messages from others that we have absorbed into our etheric body and taken to be real. This can have a particular resonance if these patterns or beliefs are inherited, passed on from generation to generation. Through the fifth attunement we are offered a release, a way of gaining insight into what we believe that may not truly reflect who we are.

Larimar is a variety of Pectolite that is blue-green with hints of white that seem to dance upon the surface. This stone has a strong affinity with dolphin beings, watery Goddesses and positive healing waters of life. Just being in its presence is calming. If we are drawn to bring this crystal into the fifth attunement mandala we draw in blissful rarefied energies. Watery forces will swim and swirl through our mandala helping us release residual tension and fear of water. If we are carrying memories in our subconscious that have their origins in the submergence of Atlantis and Lemuria, these can be transmuted. Through this our subconscious can begin to experience a freedom from ancient fears that may have been inhibiting our experience of the here and now.

Kyanite (Blue) has a unique healing role if we add it to the fifth attunement. Its energy is supremely focused and direct, helping us cut through ties and illusions that are holding us hostage. These illusions can be ideas or attitudes *which we have* that if left unexamined bind us to people and events that do not serve our highest good. Blue Kyanite combines with the fifth attunement to help us find our truth by unravelling karmic knots in the throat chakra as well as our etheric template. These knots reflect areas of our consciousness, be they from past lives or present, which have literally tied us to something.

Kyanite is a gift that serves to liberate us from illusions and fears that have their roots in our own attitude. When we welcome this crystal into this attunement we are asking to see the truth of our own mental, emotional and karmic processes that have imprisoned our own life force. We move from blaming or seeking others to change to examining ourselves, our own attitude and beliefs that have shaped who we are.

The Sixth Attunement

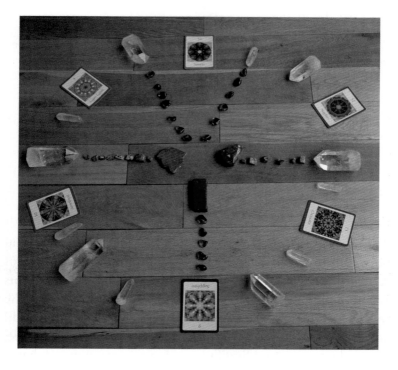

Mandala for the Sixth Attunement: as long as all the Crystal Oversoul cards mentioned are used feel free to add any or all of the crystals mentioned. In the above picture I have added a Lapis Lazuli, Amethyst and Charoite as well as many quartz points. If a crystal is added to your mandala, make sure you read what that particular crystal will bring into your attunement.

Crystals: Lapis Lazuli, Amethyst, Sapphire, Ametrine, Azurite, Charoite, Sugilite.

Crystal Oversoul cards: Azurite, Sugilite, Charoite, Sapphire, Amethyst, Lapis Lazuli.

Overview

Subject: Knowing.

Chakra Body position: Centre of forehead.

Organs & glands: Pineal, pituitary, nervous system, skeleton, eyes and ears.

Tree of life position: Upper arc of Daath.

Colours: Purple/Indigo

Musical Note: A

Seed syllable: Om

Archangels: Michael – Zadkiel

Element: Ether

The sixth attunement has its primary focus on the soul/celestial body and third eye chakra. The Crystal Oversoul temples of Azurite, Sugilite, Charoite, Sapphire, Amethyst and Lapis Lazuli combine forces to activate, attune and strengthen the soul/celestial body as well as the third eye chakra. If we also add any of the crystals; Lapis Lazuli, Amethyst, Sapphire, Ametrine, Azurite, Charoite and Sugilite, we have an attunement that is extremely potent due to the presence of these crystals as well as the Oversouls.

Layout for the Sixth Attunement

If you resonate with this attunement read the following writing first. Familiarize yourself with as much of the information as possible. You can do this process as many times as you are like. Each time will be different because it affects another moment of your journey.

Decide if you are to lie within the mandala, sit or stand.

Lay the named crystal Oversoul cards in a mandala matching the position of your body.

Choose any of the mentioned crystals or all of them. All the ones you choose will be drawn into the energetic mixture. Another option is to decide different quantities of the same stone, for example, two Sapphires. Be creative and trust your intuition. Lay these crystals within the Oversoul mandala.

Once your mandala is laid out lay or stand inside the mandala. The crystal Oversoul cards provide a gateway for the energy necessary to protect, open and offer the created space for the attunement. Relax, resting with the support of the crystal consciousness and its innate ability to transport you to the level and frequency that is correct for you. There is nothing you need to direct. The more you relax and allow, the deeper the process can become.

It is difficult to say for how long the process lasts as this work has a time all of its own. An obvious drop in energy can be felt when the process is complete.

Sixth Auric layer

Soul/Celestial — *Element:* Ether

In our awareness we travel further in the aura out into the soul/celestial body. This sheath of our being has a light all of its own. There is no known colour within the human colour wheel that can reflect the myriad of light on this level.

The astral and etheric template both serve as bridges between the lower bodies of etheric, emotional, mental and the higher bodies of soul/celestial, spirit/ketheric template/causal, star and divine dove. The soul/celestial body impresses its vision for us via our astral body. This in turn is filtered down into the mental, emotional, etheric and physical bodies, one by one. Each one of these bodies will in turn process the energy emanating from the soul plane, turning the information according to its function into action. If there is a disturbance in any of these layers, one can easily see the beginnings of energetic frictions and problems.

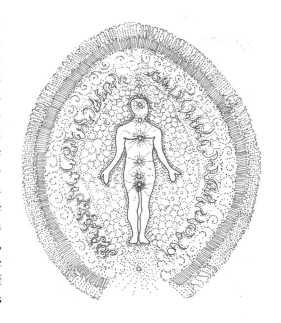

The soul/celestial body communicates to us via the medium of our intuition. If our intuitive pathway is clear and developed we will receive clear impressions from the soul/celestial body. These impressions can come in many forms; from dreams, flashes, visions, knowingness, however we receive. The sixth attunement is perfectly suited to open us to the soul/celestial realms of our being. It is a deeply nurturing attunement whereby we can experience a re-connection to our soul. Through this we can enter into deeply meditative states of consciousness.

Through the soul's eyes human life is an extraordinary precious experience. The soul body animates, nurtures and illuminates all of the other bodies via its intelligence. When we leave this world of human experience, it is through the will and timing of the soul. When we leave this earthly realm all of the lower four bodies that have served their time return back into the soul's embrace one by one.

I see it happening in this order: first the astral, then the mental, emotional, etheric and finally the physical. Our experiences are drawn back up into the soul body in order to be processed.

Some years ago I experienced dying. As I passed over into my soul body I saw all of my existence in this lifetime pass me by in a series of flashes. What struck me was what is of real importance; my memories of human contact, laughter, shared moments of love and intimacy as well as intense experiences. From this I gathered that what is important to the soul is not how we stand in society but how we have connected, shared, loved and given of ourselves.

The sixth attunement is perfect for those fearful of the dying process. Through its supportive embrace this sacred attunement helps us see life through the eyes of our soul, thereby knowing death as a natural part of the cycle of life. Through the soul's eyes human life is viewed from a parallel perspective. There is no time and space in the eyes of the soul; what happens in our perception of the past is happening in the eternal present.

Our soul/celestial body carries vast realms of possibilities to be unlocked. When I travel inwards to communicate with the Oversouls, or they come to me, it is my soul/celestial body that acts as the place of convergence and works with my astral body to gather information, thereby passing new potential through to my conscious mind to be grounded and interpreted

Sixth Chakra ~ Third Eye

On a physical level the third eye affects the pituitary, pineal glands and left and right brain functions. The pituitary and pineal glands are master glands and are powerful anatomical control units. The pituitary gland, located at the base of the brain controls the functions of the other endocrine glands, hence it is called the master gland.

Its main function is to produce hormones which stimulate adrenal glands, thyroid gland, ovaries and testes. The pineal gland is located in the centre of the brain behind the pituitary. The left and right fibre optic nerves cross over at the inner point of the third eye chakra.

The sixth attunement helps to awaken, align, balance and restore the pituitary and pineal glands to their rightful position in our subtle anatomy system. Through this process we awaken these powerful glands to enable us to see what was previously unseen and invisible. There are no limits to the third eye chakra's ability to see into the invisible dimensions. There are no limits to time, distance or space.

All together the pituitary, pineal and third eye manage the elements of a human being (earth, air, fire, water and ether). The third eye chakra is our inner eye and directs the action necessary for the other chakras to function. The third eye is the chakra gateway serving as the entrance point to higher consciousness, inner initiation and transformation. Here we surrender the soul into the spirit and learn to be guided by the grace and wisdom of our spiritual nature. This is the centre of the deep mysteries where we cross the abyss into a place of deepest wisdoms. This is the chakra point that often needs the most healing if we have been closed off, for whatever reason, to our spiritual nature.

Through the sixth attunement we can start to develop this chakra, awakening it from an ancient slumber. We awaken this divine instrument to be able to see through the veil of perception. This enables us to communicate with beings that are usually unseen by the five senses. The third eye chakra had an important role in Lemuria. It played a vital part in our everyday lives, enabling us to be able to communicate with many other life forms and dimensions. Those beings are still around us but without the third eye's higher perception they cannot be seen. The sixth attunement awakens these ancient abilities as well as releasing any fears we may still hold around using this gift.

When I write, teach or guide others to meet the Oversouls it is this chakra which is most active in me. I was born with the gift of sight, being able to see what others could not perceive. This faculty feeds into my work by giving me the ability to communicate with dimensions and beings that others do not notice. When I first encountered the Oversouls my third eye chakra was the point that was most effected, needing to expand to take in what I was seeing.

The way I came to understand it my third eye chakra needed to make major adjustments during this period of my life as it was just not set to be able to handle all the information I was receiving. It was through this journey that I began to understand the importance of this chakra in regards to my work and humanity's as a whole.

I began to explore its function in the usual seven chakra model which led me to conclude that a new chakra model was needed to draw us closer to our original blueprint. The nine chakra model, I find, supports a new archetype – one that envisions our essence as being connected to forgotten ancient roots. The third eye needs to expand in order to reconnect, it needs to operate within a larger framework that includes the crown, eighth and ninth chakras, enabling its ability to return to its original function in Lemuria.

The Oversouls for the Sixth Attunement

There are six Oversouls that create the mandala for this attunement. Two of these Oversouls are deeply penetrating in their clarity – Azurite and Lapis Lazuli are enormously powerful energies. The dark blues and deep purples combine within this attunement which takes us into the core of our being, and fears. Until these fears are faced we can never be truly free.

When I first encountered the Oversouls and subsequently wrote about them – Azurite and Lapis Lazuli held a strong hold on my imagination. Whenever I work with these two Oversouls I always think of Egypt and Atlantis. There is something familiar about them. I think that these two Oversouls have played important roles in initiation ceremonies throughout communities where initiation and ritual have played a role. That is why they always feel so familiar.

Azurite was used in third eye initiations by the Atlanteans, Egyptians and Mayan elders by placing the crystal on the third eye to help those facing the ultimate fear, the fear of the unknown and death of the self. Azurite stimulates our inner vision where we see through the eyes of our soul.

The vibration of Azurite helps us to penetrate the veil between the human world and the subconscious layers. The heart of Azurite acts as a guide, helping one cross the threshold between the known and the unknown. We gain the courage to travel deep within ourselves to the core of who we really are. Through this an unshakable knowing is experienced. The gift of this journey is a profound connection to one's intuition, to the source of eternal light, unbound by space or time.

Sugilite radiates its subtle purple rays into the emotional layer of the auric field. Emotions can be calmed and balanced through the vibrations of Sugilite, especially after shock, grief or upheaval. If you have forgotten that you are a vast multidimensional being, this is the stone to heal with. It helps us know that we are created by the same force that created the entire universe. Sugilite is especially nurturing for star children or the part of us that feels alien in this world and wants to fly amongst the stars. Sugilite will not space you out, it says 'be here, the world needs you to unfold your wings – don't fit in, let the world fit into you'.

Charoite accelerates transformation and purification through the main seven chakras. Through this process the eighth and ninth chakras above the crown are activated and opened. These energies combine to awaken us from sleep to a realized state. There is a quickening and acceleration of conscious awareness when working with this crystal, allowing us to understand our personal plan and follow the path to our deepest potential.

Chaorite enhances intuition, meditation, and relaxation as it expands the energy of the pineal gland. This gland starts to take on its higher function and operates as an important new chakra, which will take on an increasingly important role in human development.

Sapphire is an inspired luminous gem that guides us deep within to our inner master and guide. Once this relationship is established we can develop a sense of direction and purpose. Our inner master acts as an intermediary force between our conscious mind and our soul's energies. In order to connect and listen to this inner voice we need to develop certain skills. The ability to still our mind, to listen or to take our awareness to a deeper level with meditation, is needed. Through this we will start to have a glimpse into the realms of possibilities that are open to us. We will become the conduit for powerful creative forces to flow through us. This force will desire expression in the world around us.

Amethyst can remind us to take responsibility for our life force, to focus our energies and become co-creators of reality. By working consciously with Amethyst we can understand any karmic residues that may be remaining in our energy bodies. With this vibration we can be supported in facing our past and release that which does not serve us anymore.

As we shift into a new aeon for humanity, Amethyst serves to help us adjust into the new qualities of any future direction we choose to take. Amethyst gives us the opportunity to see into our future self, thus helping us adjust, if necessary, our present attitude.

Lapis Lazuli: What we ultimately seek is the truth of our own being, the power and eternity of our inner light. At some point in the life of all beings the great journey of liberation and divinity must begin. Lapis Lazuli is an important crystal giving us the strength and courage to travel to our centre. This stone reminds us that we are the masters of our own destiny, the designer behind our creation.

Lapis Lazuli serves us as a safe guide into the depths within ourselves in order to realize the peace of our essential nature. This stone helps us trust in the future, where we drive and co-create our own reality.

The Crystals for the Sixth Attunement

All of these crystals fit within the framework of the sixth attunement. You could choose all from the list and place them in your circle. Alternatively choose one crystal that appeals to you, build a mandala and place the crystal in the centre. Or choose a few from the list that appeal, placing them throughout the circle. There are no rules so be creative and trust yourself.

Lapis Lazuli: If we apply this sacred stone during this attunement we open our consciousness to divine codes. These were placed deep within our DNA prior to our descent into matter. These codes are set to divine principles of harmonics and geometry that can align our being on a deep level of consciousness.

If we choose to we can, during any ceremony or meditation, offer a release of our attachment to feelings of loss, disconnection and grief. These feelings can have a particular resonance during this attunement for people who feel cut off from their cosmic/starry families. This can manifest as feelings of abandonment and alienation which have repercussions in this lifetime. Through this attunement and our willingness to know a re-connection, we experience union with our cosmic starry family – an alignment of consciousness that can heal us on a very deep level.

Amethyst when applied to this attunement has a powerful effect on the sixth level of our aura, the Soul/Celestial body. What we experience as lack or damage on this level can manifest in our minds as loss of focus and clarity or even a sense of being disconnected from our Soul. Amethyst has a restorative quality that balances our Soul/Celestial body, helping it rebuild and protect itself. Our spiritual boundaries are strengthened, we are able to experience clarity along with a deep connection to ourselves.

Another aspect of healing where we can work with Amethyst is in its relationship with the pituitary and pineal glands. These two glands were much larger, having once played a much more important role in our spiritual template. Amethyst awakens these sacred glands restoring them to their rightful place within our energetic framework. Through this they again take on a higher awareness that reflect infinite possibilities in the creation of our health.

Sapphire illuminates our Soul/Celestial body with the highest light. If we apply Sapphire within the framework of the sixth attunement we are opening ourselves to commune with our Soul, and this can lead to deep and powerful feelings. From this connection arises a real and profound faith in our own being, abilities and strength.

Another aspect of Sapphire is its place in guiding us to the spheres of Masters. The Masters oversee humanity through offering spiritual guidance on ways of living within the world. If we choose to we can work directly with them, learning ways of being that can help us live richer lives.

When we connect with the Masters through this attunement it is our Soul/Celestial body that receives their energy. Our work is to ground their teachings, make sense of their wisdom and integrate their energy within the framework of our life. Part of this process then becomes trusting our intuition, for this is the medium whereby the Masters will talk to and guide us.

Ametrine is a crystal of rare beauty. It is a natural occurrence or marriage of Amethyst and Citrine. There is a play of colour as the rich purple and golden tones merge into one another. When we combine Ametrine in the sixth attunement we are encouraged to merge our inner heaven and earth energies. Through this we are able to see through the veil into the invisible realms yet feel our feet upon the Earth.

Azurite is one of the master crystals, having a unique place in this attunement. It is a copper based stone which often occurs with Malachite and Chrysocolla. Azurite has a powerful cleansing effect upon the human body, helping us eliminate that which no longer serves our highest good. It can strengthen our resolve in letting go of toxic energy in our life.

Through its application here in this attunement we are offered a profound initiation and transformation. We face one of our deepest fears, annihilation, loss and death. If we can learn to embrace these fears we become free to live a fuller life. When we apply Azurite to the sixth attunement we are asking to be supported in releasing these fears, to be comfortable with the transience of life. This can only happen though if we contemplate our eternal inner light. This attunement supports us in coming to know this light, embrace its qualities and understand that we are vast beings of light within a human form.

Charoite enhances intuition, meditation, and relaxation as its energy brings the third eye into balance. Once balanced and still this important chakra can begin to help us access the fine undulating energies of the invisible realms. The sixth attunement is designed to strengthen the third eye chakra with its powerful ability to govern our energetic system.

Charoite plays an important part in this process as it can deepen our ability to drop our awareness down to a deeper slower place within. From this awareness we can learn to access fine subtle information that is usually invisible to most. It is only through stillness of the third eye chakra that we can read these energies and make something of them.

Sugilite plays an powerful role in the sixth attunement through its ability to support our sense of uniqueness and diversity. As the light of our being becomes increasingly visible we will stand out and draw attention to ourselves. For many this can be uncomfortable, making us want to fit in or blend into the background. Working with Sugilite during this attunement invites the universe to support us by instilling within us the strength to stand out, be different and be proud of our uniqueness.

The Seventh Attunement

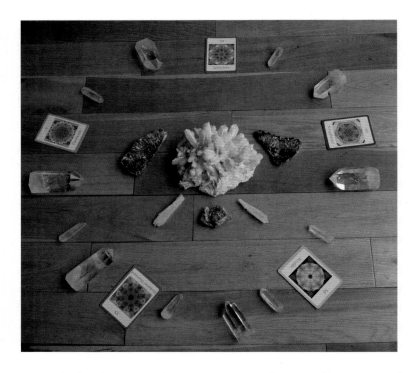

Mandala for the Seventh Attunement: as long as all the Crystal Oversoul cards mentioned are used feel free to add any or all of the crystals mentioned. In the above picture I have added a Danburite cluster, two Seraphinite, two Anhydrite and a Papagoite as well as many quartz points. If a crystal is added to your mandala, make sure you read what that particular crystal will bring into your attunement.

Crystals: Clear Quartz, Apophyllite, Seraphinite, Papagoite, Herkimer diamond, Celestial quartz, Danburite, Kimberlite, Petalite, Phenacite, Anhydrite, Selenite, White Topaz.

Crystal Oversoul cards: Anhydrite, Seraphinite, Petalite, Herkimer diamond, Danburite.

Overview

Subject: Mastery - Oneness - Alpha Omega

The bliss of union - Emptiness.

Body position: Top of head, between hairline and back of head.

Organs & glands: Cerebral cortex, skull, pineal gland & skin.

Tree of life position: Kether

Colour: White

Musical Note: B

Seed syllable: Silent Om

Archangel: Metatron

Element: Ether

The seventh attunement has its primary focus on the spirit/ketheric template/causal and crown chakra. The Crystal Oversoul temples of Anhydrite, Seraphinite, Petalite, Herkimer diamond and Danburite combine forces to activate, attune and strengthen the spirit/ketheric template/causal as well as the crown chakra.

If we also add any of the crystals: Clear Quartz, Apophyllite, Seraphinite, Papagoite, Herkimer diamond, Celestial quartz, Danburite, Kimberlite, Petalite, Phenacite, Anhydrite, Satyaloka quartz, Selenite and White Topaz, we have an attunement that is incredibly blissful.

Layout for the Seventh Attunement

If you resonate with this attunement read the following writing first. Familiarize yourself with as much of the information as possible. You can do this process as many times as you like. Each time will be different because it affects another moment of your journey.

Decide if you are to lie within the mandala, sit or stand.

Lay the named crystal Oversoul cards in a mandala matching the position of your body.

Choose any of the mentioned crystals or all of them. All the ones you choose will be drawn into the energetic mixture. Another option is to decide different quantities of the same stone, for example, eleven Clear Quartz. Be creative and trust your intuition. Lay these crystals within the Oversoul mandala.

Once your mandala is laid out lay or stand inside the mandala. The crystal Oversoul cards provide a gateway for the energy necessary to protect, open and offer the created space for the attunement. Relax, resting with the support of the crystal consciousness and its innate ability to transport you to the level and frequency that is correct for you. There is nothing you need to direct. The more you relax and allow, the deeper the process can become.

It is difficult to say for how long the process lasts as this work has a time all of its own. An obvious drop in energy can be felt when the process is complete.

Seventh Auric Layer

Spirit/Ketheric template/Causal — *Element:* Ether

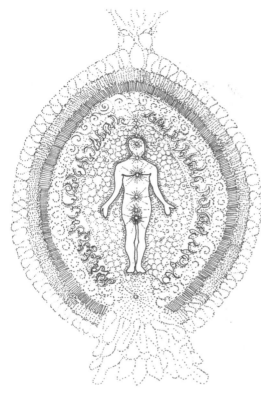

In order to connect with this body we need to expand our consciousness even further. This seventh sheath of our being surrounds the soul/celestial body with its luminous, radiant light. When a person is in contact with this layer within the framework of their everyday life the energy and colours of this layer makes an audible tone. I see and hear this layer as a vast pulsating field of golden light that streams out in all directions. The sounds mirror the golden tones like a cosmic choir singing in deep space.

The seventh layer offers endless possibilities and explorations, being a depository for all previous life experiences. It is a divine template mirroring a sacred architect's drawing, the map or blueprint of our essential nature.

The seventh attunement illuminates our relationship with this layer of our being. Through the spirit/ketheric template/causal body we face our connection with Divine consciousness. This attunement offers us the possibility to understand not only this important relationship in this lifetime but also in other lives. If we carry resentment or misunderstandings about the Divine and our connection to it then this is the attunement to undertake. Through it we can not just realize our divinity but become it.

It is through the awareness of the crown chakra that we enter the luminosity of this level of the human aura. The crown chakra serves as the gateway, guiding us inwards and outwards. We move our consciousness through the luminous light of this body to meet the consciousness of our spirit. It is through this body that we can realize our divine existence and become fully conscious of the unity of creation.

Within this body are the sacred codes that carry the potential for our magnificence to be realized. The seventh attunement puts us in contact with the overriding force that creates and sustains our inner kingdom. Through this layer we can realize and know that we are co-creators, reflecting the divine image, knowing that all is energy, but yet to be manifested. If we desire to materialize our potential into the physical world we must first imagine.

The seventh attunement aligns us on a core level of our being to an awareness of the immense possibilities we have at our disposal. This is the level of our field where all is possible, all has, and is, potential.

Our awareness at this level of our being has the ability to telepathically connect with other incarnate beings including those we have spent previous important lives with. Here we can learn to connect and communicate with others in a new light-language. We feel great affinity with others without needing to be physically near them. Space, distance and time have no meaning here. The seventh attunement will align us to group interconnections on higher planes of consciousness. If we desire to connect with other like-minded beings, be they human or from other dimensional awareness, then this attunement is the one to focus upon. This process supports us in being able connect with others without the limits of third dimensional reality.

Seventh Chakra ~ Spirit

The crown is referred to as the thousand petal lotus, as the fifty petals found on the other chakras (base, four petals, sacral six, solar plexus ten, heart twelve, throat sixteen and third eye two) multiplied by twenty make up the 1000 petals. This chakra governs the pranic energy flowing down from the cosmos into our entire chakra, anatomical and auric structure. Through this chakra we come to know that we are the microcosm and macrocosm – the dream and the dreamer. The crown chakra serves as a metaphor for our ongoing journey towards union.

We can either experience unity or isolation through this chakra, the choice is ours. The seventh attunement supports an experience of unity consciousness, showing us how powerful our choices can be when we approach fears with peace. For it is often fear that keeps us from union. When we are frightened of something we separate ourselves from "it". When we experience fear during this attunement we learn to merge with the feeling, expanding rather than contracting our energy, coming to know that we are not separate from what we fear. What we feared is no longer outside of ourselves as an enemy but an energy that once embraced reveals its gift.

The crown chakra holds the seed to the creation of our own kingdom. Thus it contains the core programme or belief that will shape our entire reality. It functions like a movie projector, and will project whatever it is we believe to be true. As all the other chakras are ruled by the core programme, the essence of this will be manifested and implemented by the lower chakras, following the nature of their role. It makes sense then that the key to manifestation is working consciously with the crown chakra.

This is the place where we heal and understand our relationship with the Divine, as well as the core patterns of our relationship with our father or an authoritative mother figure in this lifetime. How we perceive authority will be reflected through this chakra.

If we don't get our focus right at this level what flows down into creation will always be distorted. At the same time if we get the seed of belief right here at this level it will flow down correctly without causing unnecessary conflicts.

Merging our male and female energies at this point unifies and completes an ancient code within this chakra point.

From the standpoint of our human evolution we are developing into galactic human beings of light. Until we unify our male and female qualities at this level we will remain on the old template of duality.

One way of addressing this is to imagine yourself sitting on a throne during the seventh attunement. Visualize placing a crown upon your head anointing yourself as both king and queen at the same time. This aligns and marries both male and female energy streams within the crown, releasing the restrictions of the old template of gender separation. Sit on your throne feeling into your unified presence, allowing a new template to be born. This template's energy will carry you up into the eighth chakra attunement.

The seventh attunement can also help us release family and past life patterns that no longer serve us or other people we are connected with. An untying of strands of light that have become entangled through misunderstandings occurs. These strands create disharmony and inner shifts of consciousness as they unravel. However there is a point where the disharmony completes its work and an incredible stillness descends. This is usually the indication that the work is complete. As these strands unravel we are set free as well as those who were connected. This can change family dynamics as well as the history within our soul story.

At this layer of our being we can change the past, not the physical events but our attitude towards these events.

At this level of our consciousness we can experience our universe for what it is – one of many inter-connected realities that is part of a larger network of universes within universes. Some years ago in meditation I experienced a profound vision. During this meditation my awareness was drawn up outside and above my crown. Here I saw the universe that we inhabit as being joined to multi-universes. I knew from this that I am not alone in this universe. Our universe is but one of many and through the attunement of the crown we can rise up and step out into the worlds of other universes.

The Oversouls for the Seventh Attunement

There are five Oversouls creating the mandala for this attunement. The numerology of five is associated with freedom. At this level of our being freedom could not be more apt. The Oversouls working in unison for this attunement are each, in their own way, aligned to help us be free. Putting them all together creates an immensely potent mandala that starts creating the energy we need to complete the next series of attunements. We can view this attunement as preparing the spiritual fuel that will propel us onwards.

There is a particular human pattern that **Anhydrite** is more than qualified to resolve. Deep feelings of abandonment plague many people, which cause immense emotional distress.

The roots of these feelings can be, amongst other issues, residual memories from painful lifetimes. Anhydrite is a powerful healer, gently guiding us to release the past by understanding how pain can be the way that we have learnt most from. Anhydrite reminds us that we are not alone, are interconnected and embraced in the heart of the divine. What we have experienced as separation served us in reality to being guided to a deeper richer understanding of ourselves.

Seraphinite resembles the wing patterns of angels, cherubims and seraphims. It is a powerful balancer of the heart and crown chakras. Seraphinite gently and wisely guides us to the chamber of the sacred heart within ourselves. Here we meet the angels that stand as guardians of our heart's altar. This holy place is sacred as the memories of many life experiences are stored here. On our physical body the sacred heart is located on our back, between the shoulder blades. This place is where our light-body anchors its wings. If we live less than we truly are, have experienced injury, our wings may feel like they are stuck or clipped. Seraphinite is a master healer, helping us to unfurl our wings and feel the vastness of who we truly are.

Petalite is one of the governing crystals overseeing our relationship with the crown chakra. It is through the qualities of this chakra that we can start to comprehend the majesty of our own being and touch cosmic consciousness. Petalite balances the pineal gland, left and right sides of the brain, helping us bring together intellect and intuition. Petalite encourages us to seek union with the divine, without neglecting our body.

We can experience a balancing of the entire anatomical system through working with this crystal. This process creates a deep cleansing of the entire chakra system helping to release outdated patterns, toxins and inhibiting beliefs.

Herkimer diamond encourages us to be optimistic, positive and relaxed in our attitude. There is such a positive and reassuring message to these crystals that it is a challenge to remain unhappy around them. Herkimer diamond reminds us that life can be simple and easy. Their unique energy balances the crown chakra, and it is this centre of power that dictates our overall attitude to life. If we can remember that we are also made in the image of joy radiating from the crown chakra, all that manifests on our behalf will reflect this energy as well. Herkimer diamonds help us remember that we are spiritual beings having a human experience. With this in mind we see the world through the eyes of wonder and excitement.

With **Danburite** one becomes more receptive to subtle light, sound and colour frequencies emanating from planes just above the crown chakra. This in turn can create a profound sense of inner peace as we are reminded of the multiple worlds that surround us. We come to know on a deep level that all life is unified. Danburite encourages the emotional body to relax and be open to the divine presence within. As humans we inhabit a world of incredible polarities yet collectively, there is an awakening to the unity of all creation. Danburite asks us to focus on the underlying oneness that pervades creation.

The Crystals for the Seventh Attunement

All of these crystals fit within the framework of the seventh attunement. You could choose all from the list and place them in your circle. Alternatively choose one crystal that appeals to you, build a mandala and place the crystal in the centre. Or choose a few from the list that appeal, placing them throughout the circle. There are no rules so be creative and trust yourself.

When we add **Clear quartz** to the seventh attunement we are sending a powerful signal to our being. Clear quartz applied during the seventh attunement encourages us to, first of all, clear, relax and empty out dated programmes, attitudes and beliefs. Clear quartz illuminates, stimulates and clarifies our intentions. We are reminded and supported in the realization that we co-create via our intention. What we put our attention on expands.

Apophyllite serves to remind us that we are created in the Divine image, we are co-creators that seek to remember, in this lifetime, our vastness. When we work with this crystal we are focusing primarily upon the Spirit/Ketheric template/Causal body. We are offering, through this attunement, a release of attachment on our part to energy patterns that do not reflect our highest good. The seventh attunement aligns the crown chakra, awakening it to a new higher function. This will serve us well by helping us navigate our way through planetary changes.

Apophyllite is perfectly placed to support our journey through the uncharted waters of an awakening humanity, as this crystal has a strong relationship with the New Earth. The New Earth is the emerging consciousness of the planet that reflects a more unified state of awareness.

Seraphinite has a unique part to play in our journey towards wholeness. When we apply this crystal within the context of this attunement we are able to release ancient feelings of separation, loneliness and fear. These feelings are, for many, a residue from the time of Lemuria. When Lemuria receded into the ethers many were left bereft and disorientated. The pain of separation left its mark, for some, upon the Spirit/Ketheric template/Causal body. When we work with Seraphinite, within this attunement, we understand and release any ancient sorrows that we may be carrying. We can set these feelings and ourselves free.

Papagoite plays a vital role in the seventh attunement. When applied in this process it helps the crown chakra awaken to a new function, that as mediator between the seven chakra model, one that integrates the eighth, ninth and tenth chakras. Within the crown chakra are a series of ancient pathways that have been dormant since Lemuria. These pathways look like spokes of a wheel around the head. The light created during this attunement ignites and shoots along these passages, awakening us to another aspect of our journey.

During this attunement Papagoite supports an alignment with our original template, our Spirit/Ketheric template/Causal body. This can help us release any blockages that have stopped us feeling at one with our physical body and the Earth itself.

Herkimer diamond: Each of us carries a unique dream within the template of our being, an expression of our Soul that desires to be given space in this world. In order for us to discover our dream we must be willing to let go of patterns that stand in the way of this being realized. When we work with Herkimer diamond we are supported by powerful forces that desire our dream to be understood. We can, if we choose to, release beliefs and restrictive patterns from our script that no longer serve our highest potential.

We are entering a new cycle in human evolution that will require us to give birth to new dreams, ones that can only be birthed once the new cycle has begun. During this attunement we are encouraged, at this stage, to be open and receptive to these new dreams. To dream the dreams that we never knew we were dreaming.

Celestial quartz: within the seventh sheath of our aura are sacred codes, placed by ourselves in previous lives for a time such as now. These codes are carried from lifetime to lifetime, awaiting permission to be activated. They carry the memory of our magnificence. When we apply Celestial quartz within the seventh attunement we are signalling to the universe that we desire and are ready to realize, on a conscious level, the magnificence that we are. Once we give permission, through our intention, we awaken and activate the codes, signalling that we are ready to step forward embodying our magnificence.

Danburite initiates sacred communion between ourselves and the finest layers of our field. Through its vibration we expand our consciousness into an awareness of our vaster self that exists beyond time and space. We are invited through this crystal's energy, within the seventh attunement, to relax into this consciousness and come to know our inner divinity; to trust and allow this presence to guide and support us.

Through the presence of **Kimberlite** within the seventh attunement we are able to bring our awareness into the here and now. Through this, time ceases to have a real meaning or hold upon our consciousness and we can slip into a continual flux of oneness.

Petalite offers tranquility, an uplifted, expanded state of awareness. When we work with this crystal we are bathed in soft gentle light that can bring great solace. From this place of peace and calm our attachment to anxieties can be offered for release.

Phenacite assists us during this attunement by aligning us with our personal Masters. These Masters will attune and communicate with us, guiding us forwards on our journey to oneness. Our Masters work with the seventh layer of our aura, the Spirit/Ketheric template/Causal body, communicating their wisdom through telepathic means directly into this level of our consciousness. Any information they convey makes its way into our astral body to be processed and become conscious.

Anhydrite (also known as **Angel Wing** or **Angelite**) has a very special place within this attunement. When we bring this crystal into the mandala of the seventh attunement we send a signal to the universe. We are saying that we wish to remember and unfurl our wings. These wings rest between our shoulder blades. When we allow our wings to unfurl we begin to see life from a different perspective, one that enables us to be the gentle powerful beings that we are.

Selenite is a potent healer in its own right. When we invite its energies to blend with the seventh attunement we begin to experience its full potential. Selenite helps clear the energy pathways that run from our ankles, up the back of our legs, up through our spine, towards the top of our head. These pathways carry the nurturing sustaining light of our being, releasing energy into our energetic system as we need it. When we apply Selenite in the attunement process we are allowing these pathways to open up even further.

Through this our pathways push themselves upwards, making their way towards the eighth and ninth chakras. Once the pathways reach their destination they start to descend, travelling at the speed of light towards the Earth Star chakra beneath our feet. Here the pathways merge and impregnate the Earth Star chakra with a new highly refined light.

White Topaz (also known as **colourless Topaz**) is a powerful cleanser for the crown chakra as well as the Spirit/Ketheric template/Causal body. During this attunement any attachments we have to old ideas, images and impressions about ourselves can be offered for release, especially if these ideas are not the best reflection of our consciousness.

The Eighth Attunement

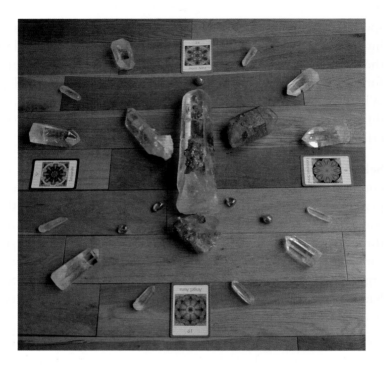

Mandala for the Eighth Attunement: as long as all the Crystal Oversoul cards mentioned are used, feel free to add any or all of the crystals mentioned. In the above picture I have added a Lemurian seed crystal (centre), at its base an Ajoite, five Aqua aura tumbles at the side and top as well as an Aqua aura cluster (main centre) another Lemurian seed crystal (top left) another Ajoite (top right) four Jeremejevite and a Tanzanite (on main point) as well as many quartz points. If a crystal is added to your mandala, make sure you read what that particular crystal will bring into your attunement.

Crystals: Tanzanite, Aqua Aura, Jeremejevite, Ajoite, Lemurian seed crystal.

Crystal Oversoul cards: Aqua Aura, Lemurian seed crystal, Angel Aura, Tanzanite

Overview

Subject: The flame of transmutation, divine seed, eighth sphere, blue pearl and discernment.

Chakra Body position: 6 inches, just above the head.

Organs & glands: Pituitary, pineal, brain and skull.

Tree of life position: Ain Soph.

Colour: Blue/Violet

Musical Note: Inaudible

Seed syllable: Aleph Etz Adonai

Archangel: Metatron

Element: Star

The eighth attunement has its primary focus on the star sheath and eighth chakra. The Crystal Oversoul temples of Aqua Aura, Lemurian seed crystal, Angel Aura and Tanzanite combine forces to activate, attune and strengthen the star sheath as well as the eighth chakra. If we also add any of the crystals ; Tanzanite, Aqua Aura, Jeremejevite, Ajoite and Lemurian seed crystal, we have an attunement that is blissful.

Layout for the Eighth Attunement

If you resonate with this attunement read the following writing first. Familiarize yourself with as much of the information as possible. You can do this process as many times as you like.

Each time will be different because it affects another moment of your journey.

Decide if you are to lie within the mandala, sit or stand.

Lay the named crystal Oversoul cards in a mandala matching the position of your body.

Choose any of the mentioned crystals or all of them. All the ones you choose will be drawn into the energetic mixture. Another option is to decide different quantities of the same stone, for example, two Ajoites. Be creative and trust your intuition.

Lay these crystals within the Oversoul mandala.

Once your mandala is laid out lay or stand inside the mandala. The crystal Oversoul cards provide a gateway for the energy necessary to protect, open and offer the created space for the attunement. Relax, resting with the support of the crystal consciousness and its innate ability to transport you to the level and frequency that is correct for you. There is nothing you need to direct. The more you relax and allow, the deeper the process can become.

It is difficult to say for how long the process lasts as this work has a time all of its own. An obvious drop in energy can be felt when the process is complete.

Eigth Auric Layer — Element: Star

At this level of the aura we start to move into awareness of layers of light that have not been visible to the human eye for many thousands of years. This body of starlight surrounds the seventh spirit level like a cloak of ancient luminous light.

Throughout history many awakened beings have been conscious of this body's potential and have used it to achieve remarkable things. By working with this body they have often

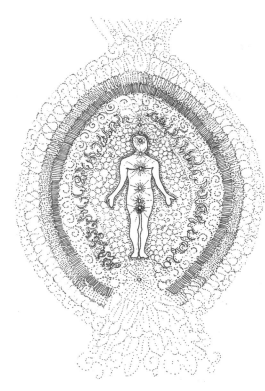

changed the direction of a nation or humanity itself. These beings were referred to as saints or mystics. I believe that the eighth layer of our aura has been in the process of awakening, either consciously or sometimes spontaneously in human beings, during the past 25 years.

When I asked the Oversouls about this they were very clear as to what is happening. The Ajoite Oversoul came forward and invited me to go on a journey. This ancient Oversoul guided me through the mists of time, and when I opened my eyes I was standing inside an ancient temple in Lemuria. I was very conscious of a ceremony taking place that involved the birthing of star beings into Lemuria. The temple was filled with the most incredible and subtle light and music so profoundly blissful that to hold my focus became a challenge. What I saw was a being entering through the top of the temple via a column of light. As the being descended slowly through the temple all the other beings present gathered around joining their wings together to welcome the incoming presence. Then it struck me why I was being shown this. The star being was entering with the eighth and ninth chakras and layers (and even more) of its field intact, welcomed by the others who protected the space for the birth of this being and its full presence into Lemuria.

Through this encounter I came to understand more of our human/star journey: also how we came from the stars in order to birth a new world which we know as Lemuria. We needed to enter the denser dimensional reality of the Earth in our completeness and the Oversoul temples existed to reassure this birth to descend through the right stages. The temples were portals, entrance points into Earth's magnetic field. Although these temples no longer exist on the Earth plane they still reside on the inner planes. There is a residue and memory of these entrance points on the Earth. These points have long been cherished and revered as shrines or places of worship. They now house temples, churches, shrines and places of pilgrimage. We still carry deep down the ancient memory of the importance of these familiar places, even if these are occupied now by layers and ideas that are hiding it.

On another journey with the Ajoite Oversoul I saw how these temples are still very active on the inner planes and transmit their energies like ripples into our reality, and I feel it explains what is happening to many of us at this time.

On another occasion I was taken into one of the temples by the Ajoite Oversoul as an observer and became aware of a ceremony. A being, who could have been any one of us, was resting in a temple surrounded by the Oversoul beings raising their wings and singing, in an ancient language, sounds of profound love. The person receiving this ceremony seemed to glow from deep within as the song and focus honed in upon them. What I saw was that the Oversoul beings were focusing on awakening the person's eighth and ninth chakras and auric layers. Receiving this awakening, I understand now, means being attuned, receiving a healing that triggers memories and thus awakens.

This is in effect what happens during the eighth attunement.

With the emergence of the eighth and ninth layers and associated chakras something monumental is happening. Vast ancient beings are awakening, unfurling and becoming present.

With the awakening and integration of the star seed into our everyday life, discernment becomes one important subject for this layer of our divine sheath. Our ability to remain open to celestial contact and at the same time discern what is of the highest light will serve us well. The eighth attunement strengthens this quality within the eighth layer.

Eighth Chakra ~ Star

The eighth chakra sits about 6 inches above the head. It is associated with the violet flame, the light of illumination, discernment, and the ability to communicate directly with other dimensional realities.

The eighth attunement acts as a balancing point and connecting force between the higher dimensions of our divinity and our human self. As we open up to receive even greater light we need to be careful to take enough time for processing and assimilating these new energies. Without this we may become overwhelmed and therefore susceptible to influences that may not be good for us.

The eighth attunement illuminates the light of discernment deep within the eighth chakra. This light serves us well as it is imbued with the intelligence to protect our life force. It has a mediating function that senses when we need to retreat or process.

When this chakra is active a light appears which looks like a violet flame. It rests above a person's auric field at the same point as the eighth chakra. It is only activated once the crown chakra is balanced and integrated. Once active, this sacred flame has the particular function to assist our karmic journey to wholeness. It has the power to illuminate patterns from our past that no longer serve us and does this by showing us, through symbolic language and synchronistic experiences, what we hold onto that no longer reflects who we really are.

Another aspect of this chakra is that it senses when we need to adjust to the influences of solar and cosmic flares. These flares will only increase in their intensity and without this chakra's function we will find it a challenge not to get overwhelmed by the power surges emanating from deep space. It acts as a valve, only allowing in what is restorative, and closing off when too much energy could intrude.

Through the attunement of the eighth chakra we can learn much about what we carry hidden within ourselves since Lemuria. Each of us owns incredible skills and gifts from that time, waiting for a sacred time, such as now, to come forward again and serve humanity. Through this we can share our vastness with no need to hide our light.

When we take the eighth attunement we begin a process of awakening by setting in motion the wheels of the ninth chakra at the same time. Our cosmic light-body descends through the ninth after the eighth has been activated. This process looks like a dove descending from high above the ninth. This dove is in reality our cosmic overself descending into our current human anatomical system. This process transforms the entire seven chakra system and thus resets it into the new template. This is what the Oversouls called the sacred point of overlap. They gave an image of overlapping diamonds descending and ascending, ever changing, wheels within wheels.

The Oversouls for the Eighth Attunement

There are four Oversouls that conspire to accelerate our vibrations during this attunement. The number four corresponds with security and stability. For me this ties in very well with this attunement as we need this in place before proceeding onto the ninth and tenth attunements. It is like we need the four Oversouls associated to this attunement to guard our energy so we do not rush any of the journey upwards.

With the **Aqua Aura** crystal comes a distinct connection to the primordial waters of creation. With this wondrous crystal we can travel back in time to the point of conception prior to incarnating on earth. Through working with this crystal we can learn to trust in our inner guidance and thus make the right choices. There are strong links to Lemurian energies with this crystal. Often those drawn to its vibration seek to re-connect and remember their power from Lemurian lives.

Lemurian seed crystal: When Lemuria receded from the earth plane thousands of years ago, many remarkable beings left their story in the crystal temples of Lemuria. These stories and experiences lay dormant and safe until the time was right for humanity to once again work within a similar vibrational resonance. That time has for many arrived.

Lemurian seed crystals are a rare variety of quartz that have ladder markings up the side of their terminations. When someone encounters the crystal that has stored his or her story a strong recognition takes place. The vibrational field of a person tunes into the crystal's memory; the story can have remarkable healing effects.

Angel Aura: one of the challenges of working with higher more rarefied light is its power to overwhelm our personal energies.

Angel aura supports us by acting as a protective valve, rather like the eighth chakra itself.

Lemurian high priests and priestesses wore robes that were the same colours of Angel Aura. When we work with this stone our subconscious recognizes its unique light. This will either make us strongly attracted and drawn to touch its colour, or if there are painful karmic memories, we may be repelled by this stone. The Lemurian priests and priestesses were known as "the Shining Ones" and that is what the Oversouls always call us.

Tanzanite: within the crown and eighth chakras above the head are seeds and codes that carry our original blueprint. These seeds and codes are often inactive and await a time when they are needed. When activated through meditation or healing, with Tanzanite, a profound awakening takes place. Intuition is heightened, as we perceive the past, present and future simultaneously; it is like having a 360 degree vision above the head.

During Atlantis and Lemuria the crown and eighth chakras were more closely linked with the pineal gland playing a more active role. The ability to access infinite cosmic vibrations, interspecies communication, telepathy and the ability to direct energies are immeasurably enhanced.

The Crystals for the Eighth Attunement

All of these crystals fit within the framework of the eighth attunement. You could choose all from the list and place them in your circle. Alternatively choose one crystal that appeals to you, build a mandala and place the crystal in the centre. Or choose a few from the list that appeal, placing them throughout the circle. There are no rules so be creative and trust yourself.

Tanzanite: when we work with this powerful crystal, within the context of the eighth attunement, we invite another stage of our awakening to unfold. Tanzanite oversees the emergence and development of a sacred seed that rests deep within our eighth chakra. This seed has, for many, lain dormant until a correct alignment of possibilities would be available. The seed once activated, through the intent of our awareness and this attunement, begins to transform into a flame of violet light. This unfolding is slow with various stages of development which will require us to be patient. As we follow the unfolding process our violet flame will reflect our journey – becoming the template for our eighth chakra.

Aqua Aura supports a further stage in the unfolding of our eighth chakra, helping us release our attachment to any karmic misunderstandings. The more we release the past and the way we perceived events the clearer the eighth chakra can become. Many people carry guilt in this chakra, which has roots from our experiences in Atlantis and Lemuria. This guilt can act as an inhibiter that blocks our eighth chakra along with ability to access the ninth and Earth star chakras. When we apply Aqua Aura within this attunement we are sending a signal that we are ready to release our attachment to guilt and wish to be supported in this process.

Jeremejevite will become an important healing ally in our journey towards wholeness. As we increase our awareness through our inner work we will of course become highly sensitive to energies. An aspect of this will be our sensitivity to solar and cosmic flares. When we work with Jeremejevite during this attunement, we are able to strengthen a small but powerful valve that rests within our eighth chakra. This valve senses energy surges and our ability to respond to them. As we increase in our sensitivity, our ability to cope with energies and flares will become more important. If we are not careful these surges will have the power to overwhelm and space us out. Through this attunement we will be able to work more consciously with this valve, being able to sense solar and cosmic flares and take any action necessary.

We can apply this in another way too. As we move through transformational times we may experience surges of energy from our own transformational process. The valve in the eighth chakra can be directed to help us stay open to any expansion in our energy while allowing us space to process it.

Ajoite assists us by balancing our inner light in a way that supports our evolution and development. The eighth attunement offers us a glimpse into our potential, shining its light into the parts of ourself that remain hidden from view.

We have the opportunity to allow what was once invisible to become visible. What was unable to be supported by the world or ridiculed will turn inside out. When we work within the context of this attunement ancient memory rises to the surface. By taking part in this attunement we are saying that we are ready to become visible. What breaks the waves of our consciousness during this ritual will be the seeds of the new – an entirely new template of possibilities that will catapult us into the new phase of our lives. What we were unable to live on Earth in our bodies, will become possible. For the first time in thousands of years our full vastness will become visible.

Lemurian seed crystal: When we apply this powerful crystal during the eighth attunement we are sending out a signal that we are ready to remember our descent into matter. Running along the sides of this crystal are magical striations. These lines are the keys to our experience as they support us in remembering our long journey from Lemuria to this lifetime. These markings carry the codes that when activated open up our memory bank.

Through the ritual of the eighth attunement, accompanied by the energies of this crystal, we are able to follow the lives that got us here to this time and place. We are able, if we choose, to release any debris we may have accumulated along the way. This attunement opens the way for the next stage of our development as we move towards the ninth attunement.

The Ninth Attunement

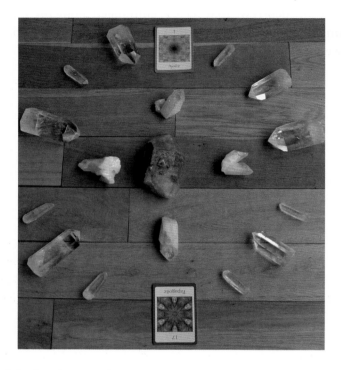

Mandala for the Ninth Attunement: as long as all the Crystal Oversoul cards mentioned are used feel free to add any or all of the crystals mentioned. In the above picture I have added an Ajoite with a Papagoite (centre) as well as four Angel aura clusters surrounded by many quartz points. If a crystal is added to your mandala, make sure you read what that particular crystal will bring into your attunement.

Crystals: Angel Aura Quartz, Papagoite, Ajoite.

Crystal Oversoul cards: Papagoite, Ajoite.

Overview

Subject: DNA rejuvenation.

Body position: 9 inches above the head.

Organs & glands: Pituitary, pineal, brain and skull.

Tree of life position: Ain Soph.

Colour: Opalised light

Musical Note: Inaudible

Seed syllable: Aleph Etz Adonai

Archangel: Metatron

Element: Star

The ninth attunement has its primary focus on the ninth sheath, the divine dove and ninth chakra. The Crystal Oversoul temples of Papagoite and Ajoite combine forces to activate, attune and strengthen the divine dove and ninth chakra. If we also add any of the crystals – Angel Aura Quartz, Papagoite and Ajoite we have an attunement that is blissful.

Layout for the Ninth Attunement

If you resonate with this attunement read the following writing first. Familiarize yourself with as much of the information as possible. You can do this process as many times as you like. Each time will be different because it affects another moment of your journey.

Decide if you are to lie within the mandala, sit or stand.

Lay the named crystal Oversoul cards in a mandala matching the position of your body.

Choose any of the mentioned crystals or all of them. All the ones you choose will be drawn into the energetic mixture. Another option is to decide different quantities of the same stone, for example, two Papagoite. Be creative and trust your intuition.

Lay these crystals within the Oversoul mandala.

Once your mandala is laid out lay or stand inside the mandala. The crystal Oversoul cards provide a gateway for the energy necessary to protect, open and offer the created space for the attunement. Relax, resting with the support of the crystal consciousness and its innate ability to transport you to the level and frequency that is correct for you. There is nothing you need to direct. The more you relax and allow, the deeper the process can become.

It is difficult to say for how long the process lasts as this work has a time all of its own. An obvious drop in energy can be felt when the process is complete.

Ninth Auric layer

Divine Dove — *Element*: Star

I refer to this layer as the divine dove. I was teaching a workshop with a large group of people on awakening the nine chakras in 2012 – it was during this day that I most understood the ninth layer and its associated chakra. Even though I have discussed this chakra in my previous written work and taught about it, I was aware that this sacred gateway still required study. I had not really been able to put into words or real symbolism what this layer really looks like or conveys to me. During this special workshop a beautiful experience unfolded which I feel explains all.

It was while I was preparing to explore this chakra with my group that something incredible happened. I was conscious of a large presence above the group that seemed to have appeared

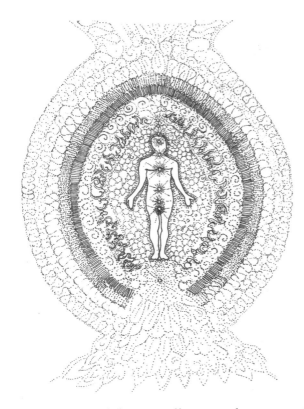

from nowhere. This presence started to take on a form – it became a vast dove and hovered above us facing downwards, focusing intensely upon the group. I knew in an instant that this was the ninth attunement, the divine dove. Although the dove was one vast luminous being it had the ability to divide itself into smaller parts. These smaller parts then entered each of the people present via their ninth chakra. This then set free the ninth sheath of the auric field which unfolded like a ancient garment of light.

As this was unfolding I understood the process of awakening more fully. The divine dove layer of our field needs to be activated within a group setting. This layer of our field corresponds to having the presence of a certain number of people willing to surrender to their vastness. When we create the mandala for this attunement for ourselves, it is the Oversouls who act as the group consciousness. Through them the attunement takes place, magnifying our potential.

Through the awakening of the eighth layer and eighth chakra we rise up into the ninth body. During the ninth attunement these layers interlock and overlap with each other setting in motion the next stage of possibilities. Once we start to become conscious of the eighth chakra and level of the auric field the ninth starts to unfurl showering our consciousness in diamond light. Wheels within wheels turn spinning us deeper into our magnificence. As these wheels turn the universe listens – for a sacred moment the universal dance of creation pauses. Consciousness has remembered itself. Ancient bells sound across the multi universes signalling that another has awakened from the dream.

The space between us no longer exists. What was separate from us is now entwined.

Our original essence is restored and illuminates our entire field with divine light. This light permeates throughout every layer of our field seeking out pockets of forgetfulness. Our DNA codes begin to rebuild, restoring themselves to their glorious dimensional possibilities. What was hidden through the mists of time becomes visible – we become what was previously invisible.

Ninth Chakra ~ Divine Dove

The ninth chakra is about 9 inches above the head and through this centre we can fully realize our divine nature. The eighth and ninth chakras are deeply connected. When we undertake the eighth attunement a profound process starts like the moving of ancient series of wheels that set accelerated energies into motion. The eighth attunement opens the inner doors that lead automatically up into the ninth chakra, setting the tone for the ninth attunement to begin.

Healing within the framework of the ninth attunement accelerates and quickens our energy. This allows our DNA to be fully restored and repaired so that we are operating at the same frequency as our first time here. By this I mean that our cells and DNA resonate with the first programmes and codings from our first incarnation into this solar system many, many lifetimes ago.

Lives spent on other star systems can be explored through this chakra. The ninth attunement is the perfect meditation to explore lives spent on other planets – just set that as your intention when setting up the mandala.

One of the most interesting aspects of the ninth attunement is that along with the eighth it illuminates an ancient code within our DNA. This code once activated sets a series of templates in motion that have long remained hidden from view. These templates are unique to each of us but they have one thing in common. They contain information that we would find useful in a future lifetime. This information could be many things of great value to us – such as the ability to manifest the tools we need to complete our task. Or the skills we would need to communicate our vision in the world. There is another even more interesting aspect to this process. Along with the activation comes an automatic illumination of the ninth chakra that changes this chakra's use.

The ninth chakra takes on a new function and acts like a lighthouse. In its new function it beams out light in 360 degrees around the top of the auric field. I think that this signals to other beings that we are awakened, ready to connect. Maybe this is an emerging function that will connect us more fully with other like-minded beings who we knew in Lemuria. Maybe these beings are part of our Lemurian family and this beam communicates to them where we are. This lighthouse beam is also a powerful tool that sees beyond our known time and space, feeding back to us information that we will need for our evolution.

The ninth attunement is a powerful healer for those carrying memories of persecution. If your core fear is that when your light draws attention to you it brings feelings of terror then this could be the perfect attunement. The ninth helps us release any remaining residue within the ninth chakra that remains fixed on the past, especially if we were persecuted for our light. This attunement recalibrates our understanding of the past so that we are free in this lifetime to expand our light into visible dimensions. Through this we only attract support from the world for who we are and what we bring with us.

At the top of our head we find a ring of light, like a halo. This ring of light is all that remains of three rings building from just above the head, over the crown chakra, then rising up into the ninth chakra. In Lemuria these rings played an important role in our ability to communicate with other dimensional beings as well as between species. The activation of these rings will play an important part in our future development, and their activation cannot be forced or rushed into activation.

Instead they begin their quickening over time, through a certain grace. Once active I notice that they not only reach up into the ninth chakra but also start to move downwards heading towards the earth star chakra beneath the feet. Once there, at the earth star, they merge, blend and coalesce with each other. This sacred merging seems to have no need to be directed by our minds.

The ninth attunement automatically stimulates and awakens the earth star chakra. The earth star, eighth and ninth are all interconnected and work together as a whole, so balance is maintained at all times. The earth star is the regulator of the entire system of the tenth attunement.

The Oversouls for the Ninth Attunement

The two Oversouls of Ajoite and Papagoite are so very aligned with the ninth attunement. On my numerous encounters with these ancient beings I have always had the sense that their consciousness is deeply entwined with our journey to wholeness. Although they have never told me directly I feel that these two beings are star beings of immense consciousness. They travelled with us to birth the earth, remaining with us until our journey is complete.

Papagoite encourages us to remember union. This beautiful crystal helps us relax and know that everything in this moment is as it should be. We are encouraged to look at any feelings that are judged as unacceptable from a point of genuine oneness. This crystal reminds us of the power of the spoken word. We can use words to build and encourage or destroy. With this in mind, Papagoite encourages us to choose our expression with wisdom and understanding. Another aspect of this crystal is that it can aid in deep meditation.

Papagoite balances both the left and right sides of the brain. Rather than these parts of the brain working apart they merge, expand and unify.

Ajoite: we are vast beings of light that incarnate, in part, in human form. We have travelled many lifetimes and have experienced a multitude of experiences to be here at this time in the turning of human history. A new cycle has begun and each of us is here to help the earth's transition into a new dimension. Ajoite's colouring and character reminds us of our ancient Lemurian light. For some, this is a painful memory as in subsequent lives after Lemuria this light was misunderstood and many were persecuted. This burdened memory has led to a reluctance to take on positions of power or responsibility.

By working with this crystal fears that inhibit the expression of our light in the world are finally healed. Our light can radiate again without attracting negative attention.

The Crystals for the Ninth Attunement

All of these crystals fit within the framework of the ninth attunement. You could choose all from the list and place them in your circle. Alternatively choose one crystal that appeals to you, build a mandala and place the crystal in the centre. Or choose a few from the list that appeal, placing them throughout the circle. There are no rules so be creative and trust yourself.

Angel Aura Quartz: what we have created through the journey of all the other attunements becomes the fuel that we need to make the ninth attunement a success. Angel Aura prepares our ninth chakra and the Divine Dove layer of our aura for an expansion of light and consciousness. When we activate and participate in this attunement we begin to awaken three golden rings. These rings above our head, require knowledge on our part to activate them. During this attunement the rings are activated, beginning their journey of awakening and illuminating.

Papagoite supports us during the ninth attunement, through its ability to repair our DNA so that it can remember union with our vastness. When we participate with Papagoite in this attunement, we are saying that we wish our vastness to come forward to be remembered.

During this attunement we can, if we choose to, remember our place in the Star Council chamber. We are guided in our astral body to our seat within the Star Chamber. Once we take our place we can bear witness to all the other beings from many dimensional universes who also sit on the council. The sole purpose of the council is to guide and support humanity. From our viewpoint in the council, through the eyes of our vastness, we begin to sense how vast, wise and intricate we all are. From our position on the council we observe humanity, the Earth and all its inhabitants – including ourselves. We feel the compassion of the cosmos surge through our veins as we understand that we are all inter-connected in the fabric of the cosmos. Each of us matters, each of us has a story to tell.

Ajoite is assisting us through helping us recall the codes that remain within the ninth chakra that will assist our development, expansion and illumination in this lifetime.

If you are drawn to, recite the following during the ninth attunement.

"Beloved Ajoite, forever reminding me of home, union with the source of my existence. Remind me of the light that resides deep within the fabric of my cells. This radiant light remains intact in a slumbering submerged place. I call on you to help me release this sleeping energy as I submerge myself in its memory. I ask of you Ajoite to help me re-pattern my auric field thus restoring me to my full divine presence. I remember, through you Ajoite, what a vast being I was in Lemuria.

I travel through the mists of eternal time and see the ancient light that never went out. As I remember union with the source of my presence I unfurl into this time and space, fully awake to my direction. The quality of my light is received by the world and I am seen without compromise for all I have to offer. My unique gifts are embraced by society as I step forward and show who I am.

Assist me Ajoite in transcending known realities so that I am able to bring my light into this temple body of mine. Let this light pour through every cell, transforming all I see, touch, and hear into an even more rarefied light. Beloved Ajoite support me by reminding my conscious awareness of the infinite possibilities I have at my disposal."

The Tenth Attunement

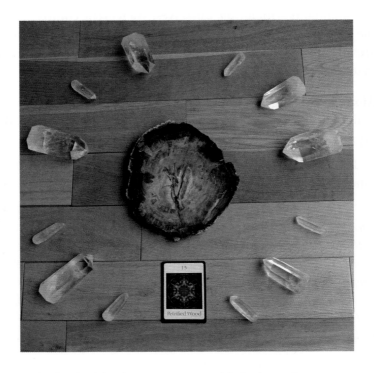

Mandala for the Tenth Attunement: this is the only attunement where there is one Oversoul card and one crystal. Petrified Wood is the tenth attunement, nothing else is needed. It is a deceptively simple attunement and yet the most powerful. In the above picture I have placed a large Petrified Wood with the Petrified Wood Oversoul card beneath all surrounded by many quartz points.

Crystal: Petrified Wood

Crystal Oversoul card: Petrified Wood

Layout for the Tenth Attunement

If you resonate with this attunement read the following writing first. Familiarize yourself with as much of the information as possible. You can do this process as many times as you like. Each time will be different because it affects another moment of your journey.

Decide if you are to lie within the mandala, sit or stand.

Lay the Petrified Wood Oversoul card in a mandala matching the position of your body. Lay a Petrified Wood crystal within the Oversoul mandala.

Once your mandala is laid out lay or stand inside the mandala. The crystal Oversoul cards provide a gateway for the energy necessary to protect, open and offer the created space for the attunement. Relax, resting with the support of the crystal consciousness and its innate ability to transport you to the level and frequency that is correct for you. There is nothing you need to direct. The more you relax and allow, the deeper the process can become.

It is difficult to say for how long the process lasts as this work has a time all of its own. An obvious drop in energy can be felt when the process is complete.

Auric layer for the Tenth Earth Star

Once the eighth and ninth layers of our aura have unfurled and awakened, with the support of all the other layers working in unison, an ancient energy initiates us onto a new level of our journey. The tenth layer of our aura envelopes our entire field. It is simultaneously deeply rooted in the Earth and open to the movement of the stars. The tenth attunement provides the support we need to begin a entirely new cycle of evolution that grounds our vast presence into matter, providing deep roots that stabilize our lightbody.

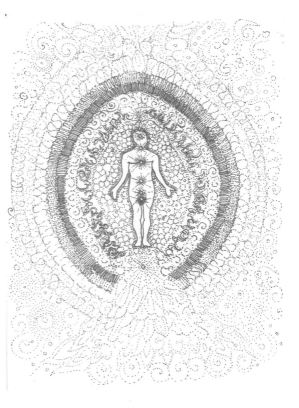

The tenth is an incredible layer of our aura that holds the keys to our future journey on the Earth. When Lemuria withdrew it took with it the support system that enabled our vast self to be visible. The initiation into our vastness is returning all of the codes and keys that each of us hold.

These codes and keys remained locked and hidden in the tenth layer of our aura until we were ready. When we undertake this final attunement we start to remember a whole new chapter of not only our past journey but what it is that we carry that will provide a part of the map of the future.

As we unfurl our vastness we begin to open gates throughout the tenth layer of our aura. These gateways link us to star dimensions and beings that desire to assist us and humanity as a whole. We start to draw towards us Star, Angelic and Devic beings who desire to work closely with us to bring about a new era of inter-dimensional communication.

Earth Star Chakra

This sacred chakra rests about 12 inches beneath the feet. The minor chakras beneath the feet triangulate downwards towards the earth star where they make contact with this important point. The sacred geometry image of this chakra is the star tetrahedron – the star of david symbol, a pyramid moving downwards with its apex pointing down, merging with a pyramid with its apex pointing upwards – a fusion of these two symbols, overlapping, creates a star of David; heaven on earth.

This chakra works alongside the eighth and ninth attunements. Once they have been activated this chakra steps forwards to take up its rightful place in our conscious evolution. The three rings of light above the head (see the ninth attunement) once awakened, begin their journey down our body. These rings have within their make-up the intelligence that seeks out the final part of our awakening.

The rings of light desire to merge with the earth star by travelling down our light-body towards the earth. Once at this point the three rings and the earth star begin an ancient alchemical dance. The mixture of all the elements that each carries, coalesces into a new energy not seen on earth for many thousands of years. The tenth attunement has waited within our collective consciousness for the right moment to come to pass. Once the earth star has awakened we start to see through new eyes. We see not just with our eyes but through our entire auric field. What was invisible becomes visible – what was separate becomes unified.

Through the tenth attunement we stand in our garments of light fully supported by the earth, ready to begin our unfoldment. The matrix of the new earth rises to greet us, showing us the way ahead. As we ground our presence into the matter into the new earth's matrix, deep roots begin to open, branching downwards. These branches seek to earth our emerging light. We anchor our vastness into a supportive intelligence that seeks to carry us into the new earth consciousness.

When we take this attunement, star and earth beings from other dimensions assist our rebirth into a new matter. These beings come forward offering songs of love that support our rebirth into the new.

The Oversoul for the Tenth Attunement

There was only ever one Oversoul aligned to this attunement. When I first encountered the Oversoul of this being it informed me that it existed just for the activation of this gateway into the earth.

There have been numerous occasions when I have used a piece of Petrified Wood, or the Oversoul card, to activate the earth star. Each time whether that be in a group, or single occasion, a different response happens. It is as if every time we work with this consciousness another layer is peeled away revealing deeper levels of our connection with the earth.

Petrified Wood: there is a chakra beneath the sole of each foot carrying us through each life, grounding and storing information. Knowledge and experience are in turn drawn down and assimilated by a larger single chakra located about 12" below them, known as the earth star chakra. Its function is retaining information from lifetime to lifetime from our earth walk story.

Petrified Wood, the guardian of its knowledge, supports the access to this chakra. Here reside the stories of all the times and lives spent on the earth. Through journeying with this stone we can explore the ancient history that has shaped who we are now. If there are patterns of fear, anxiety or pain around trusting the earth, these can be addressed and released.

The Crystal for the Tenth Attunement

Petrified wood is absolutely incredible to look at – also known as crystallized or fossilized wood – it does not actually contain wood that has become stone, instead it is the imprint of the wood that has been left and replaced by silicon dioxide.

Petrified Wood is the embodiment of all the necessary qualities that we need from the Earth Star chakra. This crystal works in accordance with the Earth Star chakra as well as the Petrified Wood Oversoul to assist the journey of our light-body to descend into matter. Through these powerful forces we are able to anchor our light into the heart of the New Earth. The energies of all the other attunements have been the fuel we have needed to propel us out of the dream, to awaken to the vast potential we have become.

Through the tenth attunement we turn ourselves inside out – what was invisible now becomes visible. We have come home, we are here in the moment. Our journey to unfold our light begins as the template of the new rises from the Earth that seeks to support and celebrate our becoming.

Attunement Elixirs

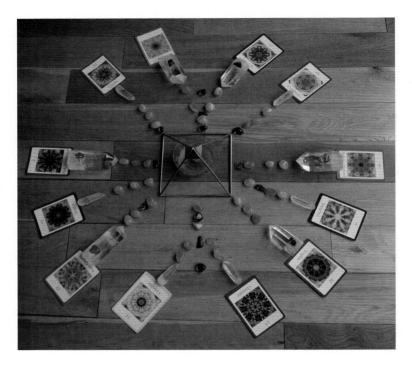

Preparing and making essences of crystals can be a special deeply fulfilling experience, as long as we follow some simple guidelines.

Attunement essences can help us release buried emotions, thought patterns and karmic memories from our unconscious. These patterns create, unless addressed, our reality. When we create an essence we take our healing to another level as the energy of the crystals we are working with as well as those of the Oversouls can imprint into water.

Water when imprinted enables us to absorb the energy required as and when we need it. All the attunements presented in this book can be made into essences. If you want to focus on one particular crystal that draws your attention or if you want to make a mandala using all of the stones mentioned, the choice is yours. When we take these essences we are clearing subtle blocks or patterns from our chakras as well as our aura. Once these blocks are cleared we can begin to experience a higher vibration within our body, and are able to express our light more fully.

Essences also serve to remind us of where we want to go, what we wish to achieve or who we want to be. They also keep us in resonance with our goal – if we slip back into old habits, fears or anxieties they can bring us back in alignment.

There are some toxic stones within this book.

I have supplied two methods for making essences. Read through this list first. If you are using any of these toxic stones you will need to use the indirect method.

Toxic stones

> Amazonite (contains copper)
> Amber (contains toxic dust fumes)
> Chrysocolla (contains copper)
> Dioptase (contains copper)
> Emerald (contains aluminum)
> Garnet (contains aluminum)
> Hiddenite (contains aluminum)
> Kunzite (contains aluminum)
> Kyanite (contains aluminum)
> Lapis Lazuli (contains copper)

Malachite (contains copper)

Moldavite (contains aluminum)

Moonstone (contains aluminum)

Rhodocrosite (contains lead)

Ruby (contains aluminum)

Sapphire (contains aluminum)

Topaz (contains aluminum)

Making Attunement essences the direct method with non toxic Crystals

Ideally make an essence while in a good clear frame of mind on a sunny day or during a full moon.

Set up your chosen attunement mandala. Place all the Oversoul cards that are a part of a chosen attunement in a circle – then your crystals around edges of the mandala (if you are using more than one). You may also want to add clear crystal points at this stage.

Place a clear glass or crystal bowl in the centre of your mandala. Fill the bowl with distilled water from a glass bottle. If you have chosen a single crystal and it fits, place it in the water (making sure it is clean.) Cover with muslin and leave (in the sun or under the moon) for four hours.

If you have used the method where there is a crystal within the water take out the crystal with a spoon so as not to add any other energy to the water.

Place this water into a stock or mother bottle. Ideally it should be a dark brown or blue bottle. Mix with 40% of either vinegar, vodka or brandy. These serve as a preservative. You can of course not use preservatives but your essence will only last a couple of weeks.

Pour small amounts of the mother essence into smaller brown or blue glass bottles with droppers. These will be your dosage bottles. As a guideline I would add at this point that you could, if you were making an essence of the tenth attunement, add ten drops. Or if you were working on the fifth attunement add five drops. Another variation would be to consider adding 17 drops, which is the number of crystals used in the fourth attunement, whether you use that many crystals or not.

Review how long to make your essence. Sometimes a few days is enough. For deeper issues you could be drawn to leaving your essence for months. You can also place drops into creams and massage lotions.

Keep your essences in a fridge away from direct sunlight.

Label and date. I keep mine in a copper pyramid.

Making Attunement essences the indirect method for Toxic Crystals

Ideally make an essence while in a good clear frame of mind on a sunny day or in a full moon.

Set up your chosen attunement mandala. Place all the Oversoul cards that are a part of a chosen attunement in a circle – then your crystals around edges of the mandala (if you are using more than one.) You may also want to add clear crystal points at this stage.

Place a clear glass or crystal bowl in the centre of your mandala. Place your chosen crystal inside a smaller bowl which goes inside a larger bowl. A bowl within a bowl. Obviously the water cannot touch the crystal in the bowl at any point.

Another method is to have a water filled bowl with your crystal nearby using quartz crystal points to draw the energy of the stone into the water; effectively creating a quartz mandala within the Oversoul attunement mandala.

Cover the bowl of water with muslin and leave (in the sun or under the moon) for four hours.

Place this water into a stock or mother bottle. Ideally it should be a dark brown or blue bottle. Mix with 40% of either vinegar, vodka or brandy. These serve as a preservative. You can of course not use any preservative methods but your essence will only last a couple of weeks.

Pour small amounts of the mother essence into smaller brown or blue glass bottles with droppers. These will be your dosage bottles. As a guideline I would add at this point that you could, if you were making an essence of the tenth attunement, add ten drops. Or if you were working on the fifth attunement add five drops. Another variation would be to consider adding 17 drops which is the number of crystals used in the fourth attunement, whether you use that many crystals or not.

Review how long to leave your essence. Sometimes a few days is enough. For deeper issues you could be drawn to leave your essence for months. You can also place drops into creams and massage lotions.

Keep your essences in a fridge away from direct sunlight.

Label and date.

I keep mine in a copper pyramid.

Epilogue

I would like to share with you a vision I had 25 years ago that has finally deciphered itself during the writing of this book. I feel that by telling this story it may go some way to explain the process and journey undertaken through this book.

It is my understanding that many of us are ancient beings that are here at this turning in human evolution for a reason. We are here on purpose. Each of us carries a fragment of our ancient story; our work is to let this come forwards, to birth and shine our light in a different time.

Some 25 years ago, while in deep meditation, a profound vision unfolded within my awareness. What emerged was a story that would stay fresh in my mind for the rest of my life.

The story unfolded in one piece, like a film, without any direction on my part. It had a beginning and an end that when completed stopped as quickly as it started. I opened my eyes after the meditation and knew that I had remembered part of my Soul's journey. It was while writing the Crystal Oversoul Attunements and subsequently this book that this experience made sense.

As I wrote both books I was aware that I was making the journeys and attunements that I was writing about. It was through this inner work that I was able to draw together as well as realize what I had seen and felt during the meditation.

Here is what I saw:

I was a tall luminous being wearing a cobalt blue cloak that was drawn up over my head. I was part of a procession of other similar beings making our way through a city. I was aware, in my con-

sciousness, that we were walking through Lemuria. Somehow I knew that I was witnessing its withdrawal from the Earth plane.

All those involved were in a state of deep peace, unfazed by the unfolding drama taking place around us. Everywhere I looked were huge tidal waves rushing towards the city and surrounding environment. Parts of the city were collapsing and falling in the rising seas that seemed to be swallowing all in its path.

We seemed to know exactly where we were heading, towards an entrance in the side of a mountain. There was an over-riding sense of rightness to our journey; as through we knew this was going to happen.

As we entered, we found ourselves in a large cave, which seemed familiar to us; there was a sense that all had been prepared for our descent. The cave led at the very far back into a tunnel that was taking us deeper and deeper into the Earth. Although I could not see the shape of the tunnel I knew that it was a spiral facing, heading downwards.

The tunnel became darker and deeper the further we descended. Our passage ahead was illuminated by our presence as a group. Our auras were emanating a vast light that illuminated all before us. I was conscious of the sound of giant waves above the tunnel that I knew must be destroying everything in their path. Onwards we travelled deeper into the spiral caves. We walked in a deep meditational state of awareness – fully conscious of what was occurring above us while remaining peaceful.

Eventually we came to the end of the tunnel. There before us opened up a giant circular room with indentations within the walls. The indentations were carved in the shape of each of us. I knew from within that one of these spaces was meant for me. As I made my way towards it I could hear the waves above become louder, I knew that the waves had entered the caves above and were making their way down the tunnels.

Each of us took our places within the indentation with our backs pressed into the walls. Out of each of us arose sounds of the most exquisite harmonies, each of us adding to a symphony that I have never heard before or since.

At this moment I felt myself dissolve into the walls just as the water rushed into the cave. I knew in that moment that I had been carrying information within my presence that I had just pressed into the walls, each of us had been carrying fragments of the story of Lemuria, to be retrieved in a later age.

Over the past 25 years I can see that I have in my own way been processing this experience and during the writing of this book another aspect of this story unfolded. It was and is time to tell these stories – to make them alive and share who we are, why we are here and why we needed to store them for so long.

What a wonderful time to be present here on Earth. Humanity is unfolding, awakening from a dream that has competed its cycle. We are incredible multi dimensional beings that have been part of previous unfolding – I am sure we will do this again and again. Each time will call for a new set of possibilities. Times that will ask us to dig deep. I offer this work as part of my unfolding journey.

FINDHORN PRESS

Life-Changing Books

For a complete catalogue,
please contact:

Findhorn Press Ltd
117-121 High Street,
Forres IV36 1AB,
Scotland, UK

t +44 (0)1309 690582
f +44 (0)131 777 2711
e info@findhornpress.com

or consult our catalogue online
(with secure order facility) on
www.findhornpress.com

For information on the Findhorn Foundation:
www.findhorn.org